Outlines of Greek and Roman Medicine

by James Sands Elliott

TO MY FATHER

PREFACE.

I was stimulated to write these Outlines of Greek and Roman Medicine by a recent sojourn in the south-eastern part of Europe. The name of the book defines, to some extent, its limitations, for my desire has been to give merely a general outline of the most important stages in the advancement of the healing art in the two Empires to which modern civilization is most deeply indebted. There are a few great works on the history of medicine by continental writers, such, for instance, as those by the German writers, Baas, Sprengel, and Puschmann, but, generally speaking, the subject has been much neglected.

I cherish the hope that this little work may appeal to doctors, to medical students, and to those of the public who are interested in a narration of the progress of knowledge, and who realize that the investigation of the body in health and disease has been one of the most important features of human endeavour.

The medical profession deserves censure for neglect of its own history, and pity 'tis that so many practitioners know nothing of the story of their art. For this reason many reputed discoveries are only re-discoveries; as Bacon wrote: "Medicine is a science which hath been, as we have said, more professed than laboured, and yet more laboured than advanced; the labour having been, in my judgment, rather in circle than in progression. For I find much iteration, and small progression." Of late years, however, the History of Medicine has been coming into its kingdom. Universities are establishing courses of lectures on the subject, and the Royal Society of Medicine recently instituted a historical section.

The material I have used in this book has been gathered from many sources, and, as far as possible, references have been given, but I have sought for, and taken, information wherever it could best be found. As Montaigne wrote: "I have here only made a nosegay of culled flowers, and have brought nothing of my own but the thread that ties them together."

I have to express my indebtedness to my friend, Mr. J. Scott Riddell, M.V.O., M.A., M.B., C.M., Senior Surgeon, Aberdeen Royal Infirmary, for his great kindness in reading the proof-sheets, preparing the index and seeing this book through the press and so removing one of the difficulties which an author writing overseas has to encounter; also to my publishers for their courtesy and attention.

JAMES SANDS ELLIOTT.

Wellington, New Zealand.

January 5, 1914.

CONTENTS.

CHAPTER I.

EARLY ROMAN MEDICINE. 1

Origin of Healing--Temples--Lectisternium--Temple of Aculapius--Archagathus--Domestic Medicine--Greek Doctors--Cloaca Maxima--Aqueducts--State of the early Empire

CHAPTER II.

EARLY GREEK MEDICINE.

Apollo--Aculapius--Temples--Serpents--Gods of Health--Melampus--Homer--Machaon--Podalarius--Temples of Aculapius--Methods of Treatment--Gymnasia--Classification of Renouard--Pythagoras--Democedes--Greek Philosophers

CHAPTER III.

HIPPOCRATES.

His life and works--His influence on Medicine

CHAPTER IV.

PLATO, ARISTOTLE, THE SCHOOL OF ALEXANDRIA, AND EMPIRICISM.

Plato--Aristotle--Alexandrian School--Its Origin--Its Influence--Lithotomy--Herophilus--Erasistratus--Cleombrotus-- Chrysippos--Anatomy--Empiricism--Serapion of Alexandria

CHAPTER V.

ROMAN MEDICINE AT THE END OF THE REPUBLIC AND THE BEGINNING OF THE EMPIRE

Asclepiades of Prusa--Themison of Laodicea--Methodism--Wounds of Julius Caesar--Systems of Philosophy--State of the country--Roman quacks--Slaves and Freedmen--Lucius Horatillavus

CHAPTER VI.

IN THE REIGN OF THE CAESARS TO THE DEATH OF NERO.

Augustus--His illnesses--Antonius Musa--Menenas--Tiberius-- Caligula--Claudius--Nero--Seneca--Astrology--Archiater--Women poisoners--Oculists in Rome

CHAPTER VII.

PHYSICIANS FROM THE TIME OF AUGUSTUS TO THE DEATH OF NERO.

Celsus--His life and works--His influence on Medicine--Meges of Sidon--Apollonius of Tyana--Alleged miracles--Vettius Valleus--Scribonius Longus--Andromachus--Thessalus of Tralles--Pliny

CHAPTER VIII.

THE FIRST AND SECOND CENTURIES OF THE CHRISTIAN ERA.

Athens--Pneumatism--Eclectics--Agathinus--Aretemes--Archigenes--Dioscorides--Cassius Felix--Pestilence in Rome--Ancient surgical instruments--Herodotus--Heliodorus--Caius Aurelianus--Soranus-- Rufus of Ephesus--Marinus--Quintus

CHAPTER IX.

GALEN.

His life and works--His influence on Medicine

CHAPTER X.

THE LATER ROMAN AND BYZANTINE PERIOD.

Beginning of Decline--Neoplatonism--Antyllus--Oribasius--Magnus-- Jacobus Psychristus--Adamantius--Meletius--Nemesius-- Alexander of Tralles--The Plague--Moschion--Paulus Aineta--Decline of Healing Art

CHAPTER XI.

INFLUENCE OF CHRISTIANITY ON ALTRUISM AND THE HEALING ART. 127

Essenes--Cabalists and Gnostics--Object of Christ's Mission--Stoics-- Constantine and Justinian--Gladiatorial Games--Orphanages--Support of the Poor--Hospitals--Their Foundation--Christianity and Hospitals--Fabiola-- Christian Philanthropy--Demon Theories of Disease receive the Church's Sanction--Monastic Medicine--Miracles of Healing--St. Paul--St. Luke--Proclus--Practice of Anatomy denounced--Christianity the prime factor in promoting Altruism

CHAPTER XII.

GYMNASIA AND BATHS.

Gymnastics--Vitruvius--Opinions of Ancient Physicians on Gymnastics--The Athletes--The Baths--Description of Baths at Pompeii--Therm?-Baths of Caracalla

CHAPTER XIII.

SANITATION.

Water-supply--Its extent--The Aqueducts--Distribution in city--Drainage--Disposal of the Dead--Cremation and Burial--Catacombs--Public Health Regulations

APPENDIX.

FEES IN ANCIENT TIMES

OUTLINES OF Greek and Roman Medicine

CHAPTER I.

EARLY ROMAN MEDICINE.

Origin of Healing--Temples--Lectisternium--Temple of Aculapius--Archagathus--Domestic Medicine--Greek Doctors--Cloaca Maxima--Aqueducts--State of the early Empire.

The origin of the healing art in Ancient Rome is shrouded in uncertainty. The earliest practice of medicine was undoubtedly theurgic, and common to all primitive peoples. The offices of priest and of medicine-man were combined in one person, and magic was invoked to take the place of knowledge. There is much scope for the exercise of the imagination in attempting to follow the course of early man in his efforts to bring plants into medicinal use. That some of the indigenous plants had therapeutic properties was often an accidental discovery, leading in the next place to experiment and observation. Cornelius Agrippa, in his book on occult philosophy, states that mankind has learned the use of many remedies from animals. It has even been suggested that the use of the enema was discovered by observing a long-beaked bird drawing up water into its beak, and injecting the water into the bowel. The practice of healing, crude and imperfect, progressed slowly in ancient times and was conducted in much the same way in Rome, and among the Egyptians, the Jews, the Chaldeans, Hindus and Parsees, and the Chinese and Tartars.

The Etruscans had considerable proficiency in philosophy and medicine, and to this people, as well as to the Sabines, the Ancient Romans were indebted for knowledge. Numa Pompilius, of Sabine origin, who was King of Rome 715 B.C., studied physical science, and, as Livy relates, was struck by lightning and killed as the result of his experiments, and it has therefore been inferred that these experiments related to the investigation of electricity. It is surprising to find in the Twelve Tables of Numa references to dental operations. In early times, it is certain that the Romans were more prone to learn the superstitions of other peoples than to acquire much useful knowledge. They were cosmopolitan in medical art as in religion. They had acquaintance with the domestic medicine known to all savages, a little rude surgery, and prescriptions from the Sibylline books, and had much recourse to magic. It was to Greece that the Romans first owed their knowledge of healing, and of art and science generally, but at no time did the Romans equal the Greeks in mental culture.

Pliny states that "the Roman people for more than six hundred years were not, indeed, without medicine, but they were without physicians." They used traditional family recipes, and had numerous gods and goddesses of disease and healing. Febris was the god of fever, Mephitis the god of stench; Fessonia aided the weary, and "Sweet Cloacina" presided over the drains. The plague-stricken appealed to the goddess Angeronia, women to Fluonia and Uterina. Ossipaga took care of the bones of children, and Carna was the deity presiding over the abdominal organs.

Temples were erected in Rome in 467 B.C. in honour of Apollo, the reputed father of Aculapius, and in 460 B.C. in honour of Aculapius of Epidaurus. Ten years later a pestilence raged in the city, and a temple was built in honour of the Goddess Salus. By order of the Sibylline books, in 399 B.C., the first lectisternium was held in Rome to combat a pestilence. This was a festival of Greek origin. It was a time of prayer and sacrifice; the images of the gods were laid upon a couch, and a meal was spread on a table before them. These festivals were repeated as occasion demanded, and the device of driving a nail into the temple of Jupiter to ward off "the pestilence that walketh in darkness," and "destruction that wasteth at noonday" was begun 360 B.C. As evidence of the want of proper surgical knowledge, the fact is recorded by Livy that after the Battle of Sutrium (309 B.C.) more soldiers died of wounds than were killed in action. The worship of Aculapius was begun by the Romans 291 B.C., and the Egyptian Isis and Serapis were also invoked for their healing powers.

At the time of the great plague in Rome (291 B.C.), ambassadors were sent to Epidaurus, in accordance with the advice of the Sibylline books, to seek aid from Aculapius. They returned with a statue of the god, but as their boat passed up the Tiber a serpent which had lain concealed during the voyage glided from the boat, and landing on the bank was welcomed by the people in the belief that the god himself had come to their aid. The Temple of Aculapius, which was built after this plague in 291 B.C., was situated on the island of the Tiber. Tradition states that, when the Tarquins were expelled, their crops were thrown into the river, and soil accumulated thereon until ultimately the island was formed. In consequence of the strange happening of the serpent landing from the ship the end of the island on which the Temple of Aculapius stood was shaped into the form of the bow of a ship, and the serpent of Aculapius was sculptured upon it in relief.

The island is not far from the Bridge, of which one broken arch remains.

Ovid represents this divinity as speaking thus:--

"I come to leave my shrine; This serpent view, that with ambitious play My staff encircles, mark him every way; His form--though larger, nobler, I'll assume, And, changed as gods should be, bring aid to Rome."

(Ovid, "Metamorphoses," xv.)

He is said to have resumed his natural form on the island of the Tiber.

"And now no more the drooping city mourns; Joy is again restored and health returns."

It was the custom for patients to sleep under the portico of the Temple of Aculapius, hoping that the god of the healing art might inspire them in dreams as to the system of cure they should adopt for their illnesses. Sick slaves were left there by their masters, but the number increased to such an extent that the Emperor Claudius put a stop to the cruel practice. The Church of St. Bartholomew now stands on the ruins of the Temple of Aculapius.

Even in very early times, however, Rome was not without medical practitioners, though not so well supplied as some other nations. The Lex 苗 ilia, passed 433 B.C., ordained punishment for the doctor who neglected a sick slave. In Plutarch's "Life of Cato" (the Censor, who was born in 234 B.C.), we read of a Roman ambassador who was sent to the King of Bithynia, in Asia Minor, and who had his skull trepanned.

The first regular doctor in Rome was Archagathus, who began practice in the city 219 B.C., when the authorities received him favourably and bought a surgery for him; but his methods were rather violent, and he made much use of the knife and caustics, earning for himself the title of "butcher," and thus having fallen into disfavour, he was glad to depart from Rome. A College of Aculapius and of Health was established 154 B.C., but this was not a teaching college in the present meaning of the term.

The doctors of Ancient Rome took no regular course of study, nor were any standards specified, but as a rule knowledge was acquired by pupilage to a practising physician, for which a honorarium was paid. Subsequently the Archiatri, after the manner of trade guilds, received apprentices, but Pliny had cause to complain of the system of medical education, or rather, to deplore the want of it. He wrote: "People believed in anyone who gave himself out for a doctor, even if the falsehood directly entailed the greatest danger. Unfortunately, there is no law which punishes doctors for ignorance, and no one takes revenge on a doctor if through his fault someone dies. It is permitted him by our danger to learn for the future, at our death to make experiments, and, without having to fear punishment, to set at naught the life of a human being."

Before the time when Greek doctors settled in Rome, medical treatment was mainly under the direct charge of the head of each household. The father of a family had great powers conferred upon him by the Roman law, and was physician as well as judge over his family. If he took his new-born infant in his arms he recognized him as his son, but otherwise the child had no claim upon him. He could inflict the most dire punishments on members of his household for which they had no redress.

Cato, the Elder, who died in B.C. 149, wrote a guide to domestic medicine for the use of Roman fathers of the Republic, but he was a quack and full of self-conceit. He hated the physicians practising in Rome, who were mostly Greeks, and thought that their knowledge was much inferior to his own. Plutarch relates that Cato knew of the answer given to the King of Persia by Hippocrates, when sent for professionally, "I will never make use of my art in favour of barbarians who are enemies of the Greeks," and pretended to believe that all Greek physicians were bound by the same rule, and animated by the same motives. However, Cato did a great deal of good by attempting to lessen the vice and luxury of his age.

The Greeks in Rome were looked at askance as foreign adventurers, and there is no doubt that although many were honourable men, others came to Rome merely to make money out of the superstitious beliefs and credulity of the Roman people. Fine clothes, a good house, and the giving of entertainments, were the best introduction to practice that some of these practitioners could devise.

The medical opinions of Cato throw a sidelight upon the state of medicine in his time. He attempted to cure dislocations by uttering a nonsensical incantation: "Huat hanat ista pista sista damiato damnaustra!" He considered ducks, geese and hares a light and suitable diet for the sick, and had no faith in fasting.

Although the darkness was prolonged and intense before the dawn of medical science in Rome, yet, in ancient times, there was a considerable amount of knowledge of sanitation. The great sewer of Rome, the Cloaca Maxima, which drained the swampy valley between the Capitoline and Palatine Hills, was built by order of Tarquinius Priscus in 616 B.C. It is wonderful that at the present time the visitor may see this ancient work in the Roman Forum, and trace its course to the Tiber. In the Forum, too, to the left of the Temple of Castor, is the sacred district of Juturna, the nymph of the healing springs which well up at the base of the Palatine Hill. Lacus Juturn?is a four-sided basin with a pillar in the middle, on which rested a marble altar decorated with figures in relief. Beside the basin are rooms for religious purposes. These rooms are adorned with the gods of healing, Aculapius with an acolyte holding a cock, the Dioscuri and their horses, the head of Serapis, and a headless statue of Apollo.

The Cloaca Maxima was formed of three tiers of arches, the vault within the innermost tier being 14 ft. in diameter. The administration of the sewers, in the time of the Republic, was in the hands of the censors, but special officers called curatores cloacarum were employed during the Empire, and the workmen who repaired and cleansed the sewers were condemned criminals. These ancient sewers, which have existed for twenty-five centuries, are monuments to the wisdom and power of the people who built them. In the time of Furius Camillus private drains were connected with the public sewers which were flushed by aqueduct and rain water. This system has prevailed throughout the centuries.

The Aqueducts were also marvellous works, and although they were added to in the time of the Empire, Sextus Julius Frontinus, curator of waters in the year A.D. 94, gives descriptions of the nine ancient aqueducts, some of which were constructed long before the Empire. For instance, the Aqua Appia was conducted into the city three hundred and twelve years before the advent of Christ, and was about seven miles long. The Aqua Anio Vetus, sixty-two miles in length, built in B.C. 144, was conveyed across the Campagna from a source in the country beyond Tivoli. Near this place there is a spring of milky-looking water containing sulphurous acid, sulphurated lime, and bicarbonate of lime, used now, and in ancient times for the relief of skin complaints. This water, at the present day, has an almost constant temperature of 75?

In course of time, when the Roman power was being extended abroad, the pursuit of conquest left little scope for the cultivation of the peaceful arts and the investigation of science, and life itself was accounted so cheap that little thought was given to improving methods for the treatment of the sick and wounded. On a campaign every soldier carried on his person a field-dressing, and the wounded received rough-and-ready first-aid attention from their comrades in arms.

Later, when conquest was ended, and attention was given to the consolidation of the provinces, ease and happiness, as has been shown by Gibbon, tended to the decay of courage and thus to lessen the prowess of the Roman legions, but there was compensation for this state of affairs at the heart of the Empire because strong streams of capable and robust recruits flowed in from Spain, Gaul, Britain and Illyricum.

At its commencement, the Empire was in a peaceful, and, on the whole, prosperous condition, and the provincials, as well as the Romans, "acknowledged that the true principles of social life, laws, agriculture, and science, which had been first invented by the wisdom of Athens, were now firmly established by the power of Rome, under whose auspicious influence the fiercest barbarians were united by an equal government and common language. They affirm that with the improvement of arts the human species was visibly multiplied. They celebrate the increasing splendour of the cities, the beautiful face of the country, cultivated and adorned like an immense garden; and the long festival of peace, which was enjoyed by so many nations, forgetful of their ancient animosities, and delivered from the apprehension of future danger." Thus wrote the Roman historian, and Gibbon states that when we discount as much of this as we please as rhetorical and declamatory, the fact remains that the substance of this description is in accordance with the facts of history. Never until the Christian era was any thought given to the regular care of the helpless and the abject. Slaves were often treated like cattle, and the patricians had no bond of sympathy with the plebeians. Provisions were sometimes distributed to the poor, and taxes remitted, but for reasons of State and not from truly charitable motives. Authority was also given to parents to destroy new-born infants whom they could not support. The idea of establishing public institutions for the relief of the sick and the poor did not enter the minds of the ancient Romans.

Before considering the state of the healing art throughout the period of the

Roman Empire, it is necessary to devote the next chapters to a consideration of the rise and progress of medical science in Greece, for it cannot be too strongly emphasized that Roman philosophy and Roman medicine were borrowed from the Greeks, and it is certain also that the Greeks were indebted to the Egyptians for part of their medical knowledge. The Romans were distinguished for their genius for law-giving and government, the Greeks for philosophy, art, and mental culture generally.

CHAPTER II.

EARLY GREEK MEDICINE.

Apollo--Aculapius--Temples--Serpents--Gods of Health--Melampus--Homer--Machaon--Podalarius--Temples of Aculapius--Methods of Treatment--Gymnasia--Classification of Renouard--Pythagoras--Democedes--Greek Philosophers.

The history of healing begins in the Hellenic mythology with Apollo, the god of light and the promoter of health. In the "Iliad" he is hailed as the disperser of epidemics, and, in this respect, the ancients were well informed in attributing destruction of infection to the sun's rays. Chiron, the Centaur, it was believed, was taught by Apollo and Artemis, and was the teacher, in turn, of Aculapius, who probably lived in the thirteenth century before Christ and was ultimately deified as the Greek god of medicine. Pindar relates of him:--

"On some the force of charmed strains he tried, To some the medicated draught applied; Some limbs he placed the amulets around, Some from the trunk he cut, and made the patient sound."[1]

Aculapius was too successful in his art, for his death was attributed to Zeus, who killed him by a flash of lightning, or to Pluto, both of whom were thought to have feared that Aculapius might by his skill gain the mastery over death.

Amid much that is mythological in the history of Aculapius, there is a groundwork of facts. Splendid temples were built to him in lovely and healthy places, usually on a hill or near a spring; they were visited by the sick, and the priests of the temples not only attended to the worship of Aculapius, but took pains to acquire knowledge of the healing art. The chief temple was at Epidaurus, and here the patients were well provided with amusements, for close to the temple was a theatre capable of seating 12,000 people, and a stadium built to accommodate 20,000 spectators.

A serpent entwined round a knotted staff is the symbol of Aculapius. A humorist of the present day has suggested that the knots on the staff indicate the numerous "knotty" questions which a doctor is asked to solve! Tradition states that when Aculapius was in the house of his patient, Glaucus, and deep in thought, a serpent coiled itself around his staff. Aculapius killed it, and then another serpent appeared with a herb leaf in its mouth, and restored the dead reptile to life. It seems probable that disease was looked upon as a poison. Serpents produced poison, and had a reputation in the most ancient times for wisdom, and for the power of renovation, and it was thought that a creature which could produce poison and disease might probably be capable of curing as well as killing. Serpents were kept in the Temples of Aculapius, and were non-poisonous and harmless. They were given their liberty in the precincts of the temple, but were provided with a serpent-house or den near to the altar. They were worshipped as the incarnation of the god, and were fed by the sick at the altar with "popana," or sacrificial cakes.

Many of the Greek gods and goddesses were held to have power over disease. Hygeia, known as Salus to the Romans, was said to have been the daughter of Aculapius, and to have taken care of the sacred serpents (Plate II).

Melampus was considered by the Greeks the first mortal to practise healing. In one case he prescribed rust, probably the earliest use of iron as a drug, and he also used hellebore root as a purgative. He married a princess and was given part of a kingdom as a reward for his services. After his death he was awarded divine honours, and temples were erected for his worship. The deification of Aculapius and of Melampus added much to the prestige of doctors in Greece, where they were always held in honour; but in Rome the practice of medicine was not considered a highly honourable calling.

Something can be learned from the writings of Homer of the state of medicine in his time, although we need hardly expect to find in an epic poem many references to diseases and their cure. As dissection was considered a profanation of the body, anatomical knowledge was exceedingly meagre. Machaon was surgeon to Menelaus and Podalarius was the pioneer of phlebotomy. Both were regarded as the sons of Aculapius; they were soldiers as well as doctors, and fought before the walls of Troy. The surgery required by Homer's heroes was chiefly that of the battlefield. Unguents and astringents were in use in the physician's art, and there is reference to "nepenthe," a narcotic drug, and also to the use of sulphur as a disinfectant. Doctors, according to Homer, were held in high esteem, and Arctinus relates that two divisions were recognized, surgeons and physicians, the former held in less honour than the latter--"Then Asclepius bestowed the power of healing upon his two sons; nevertheless, he made one of the two more celebrated than the other; on one did he bestow the lighter hand that he might draw missiles from the flesh, and sew up and heal all wounds; but the other he endowed with great precision of mind, so as to understand what cannot be seen, and to heal seemingly incurable diseases."[2]

Machaon fought in the army of Nestor. Fearing for his safety, King Idomeneus placed him under the charge of Nestor, who was instructed to take the doctor into his chariot, for "a doctor is worth many men." When Menelaus was wounded, a messenger was sent for Machaon, who extracted the barbed arrow, sucked the wound and applied a secret ointment made known to Aculapius by Chiron the Centaur, according to tradition.

MACHAON (SON OF ASKLEPIOS),

The first Greek military surgeon, attending to the wounded Menelaus.]

The practice of Greek medicine became almost entirely restricted to the temples of Aculapius, the most important of which were situated at Rhodes, Cnidus and Cos. The priests were known as Asclepiad? but the name was applied in time to the healers of the temple who were not priests. Tablets were affixed to the walls of these temples recording the name of the patient, the disease and the cure prescribed. There is evidence that diseases were closely observed. The patients brought gifts to the temples, and underwent a preliminary purification by ablutions, fasting, prayer and sacrifice. A cock was a common sacrifice to the god. No doubt many wonderful cures were effected. Mental suggestion was used greatly, and the patient was put to sleep, his cure being often revealed to him in a dream which was interpreted by the priests. The expectancy of his mind, and the reduced state of his body as the result of abstinence conduced to a cure, and trickery also played a minor part. Albeit, much of the treatment prescribed was commendable. Pure air, cheerful surroundings, proper diet and temperate habits were advocated, and, among other methods of treatment, exercise, massage, sea-bathing, the use of mineral waters, purgatives and emetics, and hemlock as a sedative, were in use. If a cure was not effected, the faith of the patient was impugned, and not the power of the god or the skill of the Asclepiades, so that neither religion nor the practice of physic was exposed to discredit. Great was the wisdom of the Greeks! These temples were the famous medical schools of ancient Greece. A spirit of emulation prevailed, and a high ethical standard was attained, as is shown by the oath prescribed for students when they completed their course of study. The form of oath will be found in a succeeding chapter in connection with an account of the life of Hippocrates.

The remains of the Health Temple, or Asklepieion, of Cos were brought to light in 1904 and 1905, by the work of Dr. Rudolf Herzog. Dr. Richard Caton, of Liverpool, has been able to reconstruct pictorially the beautiful buildings that existed two thousand years ago. They were situated among the hills. The sacred groves of cypresses were on three sides of the temple, and "to the north the verdant plain of Cos, with the white houses and trees of the town to the right, and the wide expanse of turquoise sea dotted by the purple islands of the 灾 ean, and the dim mountains about Halicarnassus, to the north-east."[3]

The ancient Greek Gymnasia were in use long before the Asclepiades began to practise in the temples. The Greeks were a healthy and strong race, mainly because they attended to physical culture as a national duty. The attendants who massaged the bodies of the athletes were called alipt? and they also taught physical exercises, and practised minor surgery and medicine. Massage was used before and after exercises in the gymnasium, and was performed by anointing the body with a mixture of oil and sand which was well rubbed into the skin. There were three classes of officials in the gymnasia; the director or magistrate called the gymnasiarch, the sub-director or gymnast, and the subordinates. The directors regulated the diet of the young men, the sub-directors, besides other duties, prescribed for the sick, and the attendants massaged, bled, dressed wounds, gave clysters, and treated abscesses, dislocations, &c.

There is no doubt that the Greeks, in insisting upon the physical training of the young, were wiser in their generation than the people of the present day; and not only the young, but people of mature age, took exercises suited to their physical requirements. The transgression of some of Solon's laws in reference to the gymnasia was punishable by death.

The third stage in the history of Greek medicine has now been reached. The first stage was primitive, the second associated with religion, and the third connected with philosophy. The classification of Renouard is accurate and convenient. In the "Age of Foundation," he recognizes four periods, namely:--

(1) The Primitive Period, or that of Instinct, beginning with myth, and ending with the destruction of Troy, 1184 years before Christ.

(2) The Sacred or Mystic Period, ending with the dispersion of the Pythagorean Society, 500 years before Christ.

(3) The Philosophic Period, ending with the foundation of the Alexandrian library, 320 years before Christ. This period is made illustrious by Hippocrates.

(4) The Anatomic Period, ending with the death of Galen, about 200 years after Christ.

The earliest Greek medical philosopher was Pythagoras (about 580 B.C.). He was born at Samos, and began life as an athlete, but a lecture which he heard on the subject of the immortality of the soul kindled enthusiasm for philosophical study, the pursuit of which led him to visit Egypt, Phoenicia, Chaldea, and perhaps also India. He was imbued with Eastern mysticism, and held that the air is full of spiritual beings who send dreams to men, and health or disease to mankind and to the lower animals. He did not remain long in Greece, but travelled much, and settled for a considerable time in Crotona, in the South of Italy, where he taught pupils, their course of study extending over five or six years. The Pythagorean Society founded by him did much good at first, but its members ultimately became greedy of gain and dishonest, and the Society in the lifetime of its founder was subjected to persecution and dispersed by angry mobs. Pythagoras possessed a prodigious mind. He is best known for his teaching in reference to the transmigration of souls, but he was also a great mathematician and astronomer. He taught that "number is the essence of everything," and his philosophy recognized that the universe is governed by law. God he represented by the figure 1, matter by the figure 2, and the universe by the combination 12, all of which, though fanciful, was an improvement upon mythology, and a recognition of system.

In the practice of medicine he promoted health mainly by diet and gymnastics, advised music for depression of spirits, and had in use various vegetable drugs. He introduced oxymel of squills from Egypt into Greece, and was a strong believer in the medicinal properties of onions. He viewed surgery with disfavour, and used only salves and poultices. The Asclepiades treated patients in the temples, but the Pythagoreans visited from house to house, and from city to city, and were known as the ambulant or periodic physicians.

Herodotus gives an account of another eminent physician of Crotona,

Democedes by name, who succeeded Pythagoras. At this time, it is recorded that the various cities had public medical officers. Democedes gained his freedom from slavery as a reward for curing the wife of Darius of an abscess in the breast.

The dispersal of the Pythagoreans led to the settlement of many of them, and of their imitators, in Rome and various parts of Italy. Although Pythagoras was a philosopher, he belongs to the Mystic Period, while Hippocrates is the great central figure of the Philosophic Period. Before studying the work of Hippocrates, it is necessary to consider the distinguishing features of the various schools of Greek philosophy. Renouard shows that the principles of the various schools of medical belief depended upon the three great Greek schools of Cosmogony.

Pythagoras believed in a Supreme Ruler of the Universe, and that spirits animated all life, and existed even in minerals; he also believed in preconceived purpose. With these views were associated the Dogmatic School of Medicine, and the name of Hippocrates, and this belief corresponds to modern vitalism.

Leucippus and Democritus, rejecting theology, considered vital action secondary to the operation of the laws of matter, and believed that atoms moved through pores in the body in such a way as to determine a state of health or disease. With this philosophy was associated the Medical School of Methodism, a system said to have been founded by Asclepiades of Prusa (who lived in Rome in the first century before Christ), and by his pupil Themison (B.C. 50). The third school of medical thought, that of Empiricism, taught that experience was the only teacher, and that it was idle to speculate upon remote causes. The Empirics based these views upon the teaching of philosophers known as Sceptics or Zetetics, followers of Parmenides and Pyrrho, who taught that it was useless to fatigue the mind in endeavouring to comprehend what is beyond its range. They were the precursors of modern agnosticism.

The Eclectics, in a later age, formed another medical sect, and had no definite system except that they made a selection of the views and methods of Dogmatists, Methodists and Empirics.

The Greek philosophers as a class believed in a primary form of matter out of which elements were formed, and the view held in regard to the elements is expressed in Ovid's "Metamorphoses."[4]

"Nor those which elements we call abide, Nor to this figure nor to that are ty'd: For this eternal world is said of old But four prolific principles to hold, Four different bodies; two to heaven ascend, And other two down to the centre tend. Fire first, with wings expanded, mounts on high, Pure, void of weight, and dwells in upper sky; Then air, because unclogged, in empty space Flies after fire, and claims the second place; But weighty water, as her nature guides, Lies on the lap of earth; and Mother Earth subsides. All things are mixed of these, which all contain, And into these are all resolved again."

Fire was considered to be matter in a very refined form, and to closely resemble life or even soul.

FOOTNOTES:

[1] Wheelwright's translation of "Pindar."

[2] Arctinus, "Ethiopis." Translated in Puschmann's "Hist. Med. Education."

[3] Caton, Brit. Med. Journ., 1906, i, p. 571.

[4] Dryden's translation, book xv.

CHAPTER III.

HIPPOCRATES.

His life and works--His influence on Medicine.

Hippocrates, the Father of Medicine, was born at Cos during the golden age of Greece, 460 years before Christ. He belonged to the family of the Asclepiad? and, according to tradition, could trace his ancestors on the male side to Aculapius, and on the female side to Hercules. He is said to have received his medical education from his father and from Herodicus, and to have been taught philosophy by Gorgias, the Sophist, and by Democritus, whom he afterwards cured of mental derangement.

There was a very famous medical school at Cos, and the temple there held the notes of the accumulated experience of his predecessors, but Hippocrates visited also, for the purpose of study, various towns of Greece, and particularly Athens. He was a keen observer, and took careful notes of his observations. His reputation was such that his works are quoted by Plato and by Aristotle, and there are references to him by Arabic writers. His descendants published their own writings under his name, and there were also many forgeries, so that it is impossible to know exactly how many of the works attributed to him are authentic; but by a consensus of opinion the following books are considered genuine: "Prognostics," seven of the books of "Aphorisms," "On Airs, Waters and Places," "On Regimen in Acute Diseases," the first and third books of "Epidemics," "On the Articulations," "On Fractures," the treatise on "Instruments of Reduction," and "The Oath"; and the books considered almost certainly genuine are those dealing with "Ancient Medicine," "Surgery," "The Law," "Fistul?" "Ulcers," "Hemorrhoids," and "On the Sacred Disease" (Epilepsy). The famous Hippocratic Collection in the great libraries of Alexandria and Pergamos also comprised the writings of Pythagoras, Plato and Aristotle.

The genius of Hippocrates is unsurpassed in the history of medicine. He was the first to trace disease to a natural and intelligible cause, and to recognize Nature as all-sufficient for healing, and physicians as only her servants. He discussed medical subjects freely and without an air of mystery, scorning all pretence, and he was also courageous enough to acknowledge his limitations and his failures. When the times in which he lived are considered, it is difficult to know which of his qualities to admire most, his love of knowledge, his powers of observation, his logical faculty, or his courage and truthfulness.

The central principle of belief of Hippocrates and the Dogmatists was that health depended on the proper proportion and action in the body of the four elements, earth, water, air, and fire, and the four cardinal humours, blood, phlegm, yellow bile and black bile. The due combination of these was known as crasis, and existed in health. If a disease were progressing favourably these humours became changed and combined (coction), preparatory to the expulsion of the morbid matter (crisis), which took place at definite periods known as critical days. Hippocrates also held the theory of fluxions, which were conditions in the nature of congestion, as it would now be understood.

In his time public opinion condemned dissection of the human body, but it is certain that dissections were performed by Hippocrates to a limited extent. He did not know the difference between the arteries and the veins, and nerves and ligaments and various membranes were all thought to have analogous functions, but his writings display a correct knowledge of the anatomy of certain parts of the body such as the joints and the brain. This defective knowledge of anatomy gave rise to fanciful views on physiology, which, among much that is admirable, disfigure the Hippocratic writings.

The belief that almost all medical and surgical knowledge is modern, though flattering to our self-complacency, is disturbed by the study of the state of knowledge in the time of Hippocrates. To him we are indebted for the classification of diseases into sporadic, epidemic, and endemic, and he also separated acute from chronic diseases. He divided the causes of disease into two classes: general, such as climate, water and sanitation; and personal, such as improper food and neglect of exercise.

He based his conclusions on the observation of appearances, and in this way began a new era. He was so perfect in the observation of external signs of disease that he has never in this respect been excelled. The state of the face, eyes, tongue, voice, hearing, abdomen, sleep, breathing, excretions, posture of the body, and so on, all aided him in diagnosis and prognosis, and to the latter he paid special attention, saying that "the best physician is the one who is able to establish a prognosis, penetrating and exposing first of all, at the bedside, the present, the past, and the future of his patients, and adding what they omit in their statements. He gains their confidence, and being convinced of his superiority of knowledge they do not hesitate to commit themselves entirely into his hands. He can treat, also, so much better their present condition in proportion as he shall be able from it to foresee the future."

He wrote about the history of Medicine, a study which is much neglected at the present time. There is no generation of men so wise that they cannot with advantage adopt some ideas from the remote past, or, at least, find the teaching of their predecessors suggestive. Hippocrates was one of the first to recognize the vis medicatrix natur? and he always aimed at assisting Nature. His style of treatment would be known now as expectant, and he tried to order his practice "to do good, or, at least, to do no harm." When he considered interference necessary, however, he did not hesitate even to apply drastic measures, such as scarification, cupping and bleeding. He made use of the narcotics mandragora, henbane, and probably also poppy-juice, and as a laxative used greatly a vegetable substance called "mercury," beet and cabbage, and cathartics such as scammony and elaterium! He was able to diagnose fluid in the chest or abdomen by means of percussion and auscultation, and to withdraw the fluid by the operation of paracentesis, and he recognized also that the fluid should be allowed to flow away slowly so as to minimize the risk of syncope. He operated also for empyema. In regard to the methods of Hippocrates for the physical examination of the chest it is reasonable to suppose that the Father of Medicine indirectly inspired Laennec to invent the stethoscope. Hippocrates prescribed fluid diet for fevers, allowed the patients cold water or barley water to drink, and recommended cold sponging for high fever. In his writings will be found his views on apoplexy, epilepsy, phthisis, gout, erysipelas, cancer and many other diseases common at the present day.

In the province of Surgery, Hippocrates was surprisingly proficient, although he lived before the Anatomic Period. He had various lotions for the healing of ulcers; some of these lotions were antiseptic and have been in use in recent times. His opinions on the treatment of fractures are sound, and he was a master in the use of splints, and considered that it was disgraceful on the part of the surgeon to allow a broken limb to set in a faulty position. He resected the projecting ends of the bone in the case of compound fracture. He had a very complete knowledge of the anatomy of joints, was well acquainted with hip-joint disease, and could operate upon joints. Accidents were no doubt common in the gymnasia, and practice in the treatment of fractures and dislocations extensive and of a high order of excellence. Hippocrates used the sound for exploring the bladder, and understood the use of the speculum for examining the rectum, and in operations for fistula and piles. He understood the causation of club-foot, and could cure cases of this deformity by bandaging. He was skilful also in obstetric operations. He trepanned the skull, which appears to have been a common operation in his day. He had clear and sound views in reference to wounds of the head, recognizing that trivial-looking wounds of the scalp might become very serious. Hippocrates gave directions as to the indications for using the trepan, and warned the operator against mistaking sutures of the cranial bones for fracture.

He did not describe amputations as generally understood, but removed limbs at a joint for gangrene. When necessary he made use of mechanical appliances for reducing dislocations, and recommended doctors to furnish their surgeries with an adjustable table, fitted with levers, for dealing with the reduction of dislocations, and for various other surgical manipulations. Excision of tumours was not a common operation of Hippocratic surgery, although it had been a part of Hindu practice in very ancient times. On the subject of Obstetrics, Hippocrates wrote a great deal, and although many of his theories seem absurd at the present day, yet, on the whole, the treatment he recommends is efficacious. Regarding Gynecology, in his treatise on "Airs, Water and Places," it is interesting to observe that he says that the drinking of impure water will cause dropsy of the uterus. Adams, commenting on this, has in mind hydatids, but it is evident that both Hippocrates and his translator and critic have mistaken hydatidiform disease of the ovum for hydatid disease of the womb. In the books which are considered genuine the references to diseases of women are meagre, and it is likely that the author had little special knowledge of the subject. That part of the Hippocratic collection which is not considered genuine deals rather fully with the subject of gynecology.[5] In it are described sounds made of wood and of lead, dilators and uterine catheters. Sitz baths were in use, and fumigations were very extensively employed in gynecological practice. Pessaries were made by rolling lint or wool into an oblong shape, and were medicated to be emollient, astringent or purgative in their local action. The half of a pomegranate was used as a mechanical pessary, and there are also references to tents, and to suppositories for the bowel.

In dealing with Dietetics, Hippocrates displays close observation and sound judgment. The views held generally at the present day coincide closely with his instructions on food and feeding. In the treatise on Ancient Medicine, he states that men had to find from experience the properties of various vegetable foods, and discovered that what was suitable in health was unsuitable in sickness, and that the accumulation of these discoveries was the origin of the art of medicine.

The Sydenham Society initiated, and Dr. Adams brilliantly accomplished, a noble work in the publication in 1849 of "The Genuine Works of Hippocrates," from which "The Law," and "The Oath" are here quoted. The former is the view of Hippocrates of the standards which should govern the practice of medicine; the latter is that by which all the Aculapians were bound.

"THE LAW.

"(1) Medicine is of all the arts the most noble; but, owing to the ignorance of those who practise it, and of those who, inconsiderately, form a judgment of them, it is at present far behind all the other arts. Their mistake appears to me to arise principally from this, that in the cities there is no punishment connected with the practice of medicine (and with it alone) except disgrace, and that does not hurt those who are familiar with it. Such persons are like the figures which are introduced in tragedies, for as they have the shape, and dress, and personal appearance of an actor, but are not actors, so also physicians are many in title but very few in reality.

"(2) Whoever is to acquire a competent knowledge of medicine, ought to be possessed of the following advantages: A natural disposition; instruction; a favourable position for the study; early tuition; love of labour; leisure. First of all, a natural talent is required, for, when Nature opposes, everything else is vain; but when Nature leads the way to what is most excellent, instruction in the art takes place, which the student must try to appropriate to himself by reflection, becoming an early pupil in a place well adapted for instruction. He must also bring to the task a love of labour and perseverance, so that the instruction taking root may bring forth proper and abundant fruits.

"(3) Instruction in medicine is like the culture of the productions of the earth. For our natural disposition is, as it were, the soil; the tenets of our teacher are, as it were, the seed; instruction in youth is like the planting of the seed in the ground at the proper season; the place where the instruction is communicated is like the food imparted to vegetables by the atmosphere; diligent study is like the cultivation of the fields; and it is time which imparts strength to all things and brings them to maturity.

"(4) Having brought all these requisites to the study of medicine, and having acquired a true knowledge of it, we shall thus, in travelling through the cities, be esteemed physicians not only in name but in reality. But inexperience is a bad treasure, and a bad friend to those who possess it, whether in opinion or reality, being devoid of self-reliance and contentedness, and the nurse both of timidity and audacity. For timidity betrays a want of powers, and audacity a want of skill. There are, indeed, two things, knowledge and opinion, of which the one makes its possessor really to know, the other to be ignorant.

"(5) These things which are sacred are to be imparted only to sacred persons;

and it is not lawful to impart them to the profane until they have been initiated in the mysteries of the science."

"THE OATH.

"I swear by Apollo, the physician, and Aculapius, and Health, and Panacea, and all the gods and goddesses, that, according to my ability and judgment, I will keep this oath and this stipulation--to reckon him who taught me this art equally dear to me as my parents, to share my substance with him, and relieve his necessities if required; to look upon his offspring in the same footing as my own brothers, and to teach them this art, if they shall wish to learn it, without fee or stipulation; and that by precept, lecture, and every other mode of instruction, I will impart a knowledge of the Art to my own sons, and those of my teachers, and to disciples bound by a stipulation and oath according to the law of medicine, but to none others. I will follow that system of regimen which, according to my ability and judgment, I consider for the benefit of my patients, and abstain from whatever is deleterious and mischievous. I will give no deadly medicine to anyone if asked, nor suggest any such counsel; and in like manner I will not give to a woman a pessary to produce abortion. With purity and with holiness I will pass my life and practise my Art. I will not cut persons labouring under the stone, but will leave this to be done by men who are practitioners of this work. Into whatever houses I enter, I will go into them for the benefit of the sick, and will abstain from every voluntary act of mischief and corruption, and, further, from the seduction of females or males, of freedmen and slaves. Whatever, in connection with my professional practice, or not in connection with it, I see or hear, in the life of men, which ought not to be spoken of abroad, I will not divulge as reckoning that all such should be kept secret. While I continue to keep this Oath inviolate, may it be granted to me to enjoy life and the practice of the Art, respected by all men, in all times! But should I trespass or violate this oath, may the reverse be my lot!"

It would be a great task to attempt anything like a full review of the writings of this great doctor of antiquity, but enough has been written to reveal the great powers of his mind, and to show that he was far in advance of his predecessors, and a model for his successors. In the island of Cos, made illustrious by the name of Hippocrates, it is strange to find that he has no fame now other than that of being regarded in the confused minds of the people as one of the numerous saints of the Greek Church.[6]

"When," says Littr? "one searches into the history of medicine and the commencement of science, the first body of doctrine that one meets with is the collection of writings known under the name of the works of Hippocrates. The science mounts up directly to that origin, and there stops. Not that it had not been cultivated earlier, and had not given rise to even numerous productions; but everything that had been made before the physician of Cos has perished. We have only remaining of them scattered and unconnected fragments. The works of Hippocrates have alone escaped destruction; and by a singular circumstance there exists a great gap after them as well as before them. The medical works from Hippocrates to the establishment of the School of Alexandria, and those of that school itself, are completely lost, except some quotations and passages preserved in the later writers; so that the writings of Hippocrates remain alone amongst the ruins of ancient medical literature." Sydenham said of Hippocrates: "He it is whom we can never duly praise," and refers to him as "that divine old man," and "the Romulus of medicine, whose heaven was the empyrean of his art."

Hippocrates died in Thessaly, but at what age is uncertain, for different authors have credited him with a lifetime of from eighty-five to a hundred and nine years. By virtue of his fame, death for him was not the Great Leveller.

Hippocrates had two sons, Thessalus and Draco; the former was physician to Archelaus, King of Macedonia, the latter physician to the wife of Alexander the Great. They were the founders of the School of Dogmatism which was based mainly on the teaching and aphorisms of Hippocrates. The Dogmatic Sect emphasized the importance of investigating not the obvious but the underlying and hidden causes of disease and held undisputed sway until the foundation of the Empirical Sect at Alexandria.

FOOTNOTES:

[5] Vide "History of Gynecology," by W. J. Stewart McKay. Baillie, Tindall and Cox, 1901.

[6] Archiv Geschichte der Medizin, May, 1912.

CHAPTER IV.

PLATO, ARISTOTLE, THE SCHOOL OF ALEXANDRIA AND EMPIRICISM.

Plato--Aristotle--Alexandrian School--Its Origin--Its Influence-- Lithotomy--Herophilus--Erasistratus--Cleombrotus--Chrysippos-- Anatomy--Empiricism--Serapion of Alexandria.

Two very eminent philosophers, Plato and Aristotle, were influenced by the teaching of Hippocrates.

Plato (B.C. 427-347) was a profound moralist, and though possessed of one of the keenest intellects of all time, did little to advance medical science. He did not practise medicine, but studied it as a branch of philosophy, and instead of observing and investigating, attempted to solve the problems of health and disease by intuition and speculation. His conceptions were inaccurate and fantastic.

He elaborated the humoral pathology of Hippocrates. The world, he thought, was composed of four elements: fire consisting of pyramidal, earth of cubical, air of octagonal, and water of twenty-sided atoms. The marrow consists of triangles, and the brain is the perfection of marrow. The soul dominates the marrow and the separation of the two causes death. The purpose of the bones and muscles is to protect the marrow against changes of temperature. Plato divided the "soul" into three parts: Reason, enthroned in the brain;

courage in the heart; and desire in the liver. The uterus, he believed, excites inordinate desires. Inflammations are due to disorders of the bile, and fevers to the influence of the elements. His theories in regard to the special senses are very fantastic, for instance, smell is evanescent because it is not founded on any external image; taste results from small vessels carrying taste atoms to the heart and soul.

Aristotle, born B.C. 334, was the son of Nichomachus, physician to the King of Macedonia, and of the race of the Asclepiads. His inherited taste was for the study of Nature; he attained the great honour of being the founder of the sciences of Comparative Anatomy and Natural History, and contributed largely to the medical knowledge of his time. Aristotle went to Athens and became a follower of Plato, and the close companionship of these two great men lasted for twenty years. At the age of 42, Aristotle was appointed by Philip of Macedon tutor to Alexander the Great, who was then aged 15, and the interest of that mighty prince was soon aroused in the study of Natural History. Aristotle and Alexander the Great, teacher and pupil, founded the first great Natural History Museum, to which specimens were sent from places scattered over the then known world. Aristotle, besides his philosophical books, wrote: "Researches about Animals," "On Sleep and Waking," "On Longevity and Shortlivedness," "On Parts of Animals," "On Respiration," "On Locomotion of Animals," and "On Generation of Animals." He was greatly helped in the supply of material for dissection in his study of comparative anatomy by his pupil, Alexander the Great. Aristotle pointed out the differences in the anatomy of men and monkeys; he described the anatomy of the elephant and of birds, and also the changes in development seen during the incubation of eggs. He investigated, also, the anatomy of fishes and reptiles. The stomachs of ruminant animals excited his interest, and he described their structure. The heart, according to Aristotle, was the seat of the soul, and the birthplace of the passions, for it held the natural fire, and in it centred movement, sensation and nourishment. The diaphragm, he believed, separated the heart, the seat of the soul, from the contaminating influences of the intestines. He did not advance beyond the conception that nerves were akin to ligaments and tendons, and he believed that the nerves originated in the heart, as did also the blood-vessels. He named the aorta and ventricles. He investigated the action of the muscles, and held that superfoetation was possible.

When Aristotle retired to Chalcis, he chose Tyrtamus, to whom he gave the name of Theophrastus, as his successor at the Lyceum. Theophrastus was the originator of the science of Botany, and wrote the "History of Plants." He also wrote about stones, and on physical, moral and medical subjects.

THE ALEXANDRIAN SCHOOL.

"In the year 331 B.C.," wrote Kingsley, "one of the greatest intellects whose influence the world has ever felt, saw, with his eagle glance, the unrivalled advantages of the spot which is now Alexandria, and conceived the mighty project of making it the point of union of two, or rather of three worlds. In a new city named after himself, Europe, Asia and Africa were to meet and hold communion." The School of Alexandria became, after the decay of Greek culture, the centre of learning for the world, and when the Empire of Alexander the Great was subdivided, the Egyptian share fell to the first Ptolemy, who, under the direction of Aristotle, founded the Alexandrian Library, containing at first fifty thousand, and finally seven hundred thousand volumes. Every student who came to the University of Alexandria, and possessed a book of which there was not a copy in the Alexandrian Library, was compelled to present the book to the library. The first Ptolemy also fostered the study of medicine and of dissection. Eumenes likewise established a library at Pergamos. It is instructive to follow the history of the great Library of Alexandria. The greater part of the library, which contained the collected literature of Greece, Rome, India and Egypt, was housed in the famous museum in the part of Alexandria called the Brucheion. This part was destroyed by fire during the siege of Alexandria by Julius Caesar. Mark Antony, then, at the urgent desire of Cleopatra, transferred to Alexandria the books and manuscripts from Pergamos. The other part of the library was kept at Alexandria in the Serapeum, the temple of Jupiter Serapis, and there it remained till the time of Theodosius the Great, until in 391 A.D. both temple and library were almost completely destroyed by a fanatical mob of Christians led by the Archbishop Theophilus. When Alexandria was taken by the Arabs in 641, under the Calif Omar, the destruction was completed.

Ptolemy gathered to the museum at Alexandria a number of very learned men, who lived within its walls and were provided with salaries, the whole system closely resembling a university. Grammar, prosody, mythology, astronomy and philosophy were studied, and great attention was given to the study of medicine. Euclid was the teacher of Mathematics, and Hipparchus of Alexandria was the father of Astronomy. The teaching of medicine and of astronomy was for long based upon observation of ascertained facts. The Alexandrian School endured for close upon a thousand years, and its history may be divided into two periods, namely, from 323 to 30 B.C., during the period of the Ptolemies, and from 30 B.C. to 640 A.D. The second period was distinguished for the study of speculative philosophy, and of the religious philosophy of the Gnostics, and was not a scientific period.

Julius Caesar was not the only Roman Emperor who brought trouble upon the Alexandrian School, for the brutal Caracalla took away the salaries and privileges from the savants, and prohibited scientific exhibitions and discussions. In recent excavations in the Baths of Caracalla in Rome, the ruins of a library have been discovered, and it is believed by some archelogists that Caracalla supplied this library with books and parchments from Alexandria.

The Asclepiad?of Cos and Cnidos had discoursed upon the phenomena of disease, without attempting to demonstrate its structural relations; like the sculptors of their own age, they studied the changing expression of vital action almost wholly from an external point of view. They meddled not with the dead, for, by their own laws, no one was allowed to die within the temple. But the early Alexandrians were subject to no such restrictions; and turning to good account the discoveries of Aristotle in natural history and comparative anatomy, they undertook for the first time to describe the organization of the human frame from actual dissections.[7]

Thus there was inaugurated at Alexandria the Anatomic Period of Medicine, which lasted till Egypt came under the sway of the Romans. Medical practice became so flourishing at Alexandria that three great specialities were established, namely, Surgery, Pharmacy, and Dietetics, and a great variety of operations were performed. Lithotomy was much practised by specialists. A foul murder was perpetrated by lithotomists at the instigation of Diodotus, the guardian of Antiochus, son of Alexander, King of Syria (150 B.C.), young Antiochus, at the age of 10, being done to death under the pretence that he had a stone in his bladder.

About 150 B.C. a sect called the Essenes was established for the study of curative and poisonous substances. The members were not all physicians, by any means, for one of the chief was King Mithridates, who invented the remedy known as mithridaticum. This celebrated nostrum of antiquity is said to have been a confection of twenty leaves of rue, a few grains of salt, two walnuts, and two figs, intended to be taken every morning and followed by a draught of wine.

Two famous physicians and anatomists, Herophilus (335-280 B.C.) and Erasistratus (280 B.C.) took part in the medical teaching at Alexandria in the early days of that seat of learning. It is recorded that they did not confine their investigations to the dissection of the dead, but also vivisected criminals. Cleombrotus, another physician at this school, was sent for to attend King Antiochus, and was rewarded with a hundred talents, equal to about ?5,000 sterling.

There were several physicians of the name of Chrysippos connected with the Alexandrian School. One was physician to Ptolemy Soter, the King of Egypt, and tutor to Erasistratus. This Chrysippos introduced the practice of emptying a limb of blood before amputation, according to the recent method of Esmarch, and is said to have employed vapour baths in the treatment of dropsy.

In Alexandria, anatomy was properly studied.[8]

Herophilus made many anatomical discoveries, and some of the names he gave to parts of the body are now in use, for instance, torcular Herophili, calamus scriptorius, and duodenum. He described the connection between the nerves and the brain, and the various parts of the brain, and recognized the essential difference between motor and sensory nerves, although he thought the former arose in the membranes and the latter in the substance of the brain. He believed that the fourth ventricle was the seat of the soul. He attributed to the heart the pulsations of the arteries, but thought that the pulmonary veins conveyed air from the lungs to the left side of the heart, and he observed the lacteals without determining their function. Herophilus operated upon the liver and spleen, and looked upon the latter as of little consequence in the animal economy. He had a good knowledge of obstetric operations. His ideas in relation to pathology did not proceed much further than the belief that disease was due to corruption of the humors. He was more scientific and accurate when he taught that paralysis results from a defect in the nerves.

Erasistratus studied under Chrysippos (or Chrysippus), and under Metrodorus, the son-in-law of Aristotle. Herophilus had been a student at Cos, Erasistratus at Cnidos, so that the teaching of the two great Greek medical schools was introduced into Alexandria. Xenophon, of Cos, one of the followers of Erasistratus, first resorted to the ligation of vessels for the arrest of h鎚orrhage, although for many years in later times this important practice was lost through the neglect of the study of the history of medicine. Erasistratus and Herophilus, it is sad to relate, considered that vivisection of human beings, as well as dissection of the dead, was a necessary part of medical education, and believed that the sufferings of a few criminals did not weigh against the benefit likely to accrue to innocent people, who could be relieved or cured of disease and suffering as the result of the knowledge gained by dissection of the living. This cruel and nefarious practice was followed "so that the investigators could study the particular organs during life in regard to position, colour, form, size, disposition, hardness, softness, smoothness, and superficial extent, their projection and curvatures."

The followers of these teachers, unfortunately, became very speculative and fond of discussions of a fruitless kind, and, according to Pliny, it was easier "to sit and listen quietly in the schools than to be up and wandering over the deserts, and to seek out new plants every day,"[9] and so, in the third century before Christ, the school of Empiricism was established, the system of which resembled the older Scepticism. It rested upon the "Empiric tripod," namely, accident, history and analogy. This meant that discoveries were made by accident, knowledge was accumulated by the recollection of previous cases, and treatment adopted which had been found suitable in similar circumstances. Philinus of Cos, a pupil of Herophilus, declared that all the anatomy he had learned from his master did not help him in the least to cure diseases. Philinus, according to Galen, founded the Empirici, the first schismatic sect in medicine. Celsus[10] wrote of this sect that they admit that evident causes are necessary, but deprecate inquiry into them because Nature is incomprehensible. This is proved because the philosophers and physicians who have spent so much labour in trying to search out these occult causes cannot agree amongst themselves. If reasoning could make physicians, the philosophers should be most successful practitioners, as they have such abundance of words. If the causes of diseases were the same in all places, the same remedies ought to be used everywhere. Relief from sickness is to be sought from things certain and tried, that is from experience, which guides us in all other arts. Husbandmen and pilots do not reason about their business, but they practise it. Disquisitions can have no connection with medicine, because physicians whose opinions have been directly opposed to one another have equally restored their patients to health; they did not derive their methods of cure from studying the occult causes about which they disputed, but from the experience they had of the remedies which they employed upon their patients. Medicine was not first discovered in consequence of reasoning, but the theory was sought for after the discovery of medicine. Does reason, they ask, prescribe the same as experience, or something different? If the same, it must be needless; if different, it must be mischievous.

In the third and second centuries before Christ, many physicians wrote commentaries on diseases and attacked the teaching of Hippocrates. Among these, Serapion of Alexandria, an Empiric who lived in the third century before Christ, is noteworthy for having first used sulphur in the treatment of skin diseases, and Heraclides wrote on strangulated hernia. Serapion added somewhat to the system of Philinus, and was responsible for introducing the principle of analogy into the system of Empiricism. The foundation of Empiricism marked the decline of the medical school of Alexandria. We are indebted to Celsus for a full description of the teaching of this sect, and, at the same time, for an exposure of its fallacies. Serapion was a convert from the school of Cos, which was the stronghold of medical dogmatism, and, like nearly all apostates, he was consumed with animosity and bitterness towards those with whom he had formerly been in agreement. Cnidos was the stronghold of the Empirics.

FOOTNOTES:

[7] "The Medical Profession in Ancient Times." Watson, p. 90.

[8] Arctinus: "Ethiopis," Translated in Puschmann's "Hist. Med. Education."

[9] Pliny, "Hist. Nat.," xxvi, 6.

[10] "De Med.," Prat. (Translation.)

CHAPTER V.

ROMAN MEDICINE AT THE END OF THE REPUBLIC AND THE BEGINNING OF THE EMPIRE.

Asclepiades of Prusa--Themison of Laodicea--Methodism--Wounds of Julius Caesar--Systems of Philosophy--State of the country--Roman quacks--Slaves and Freedmen--Lucius Horatillavus.

Asclepiades of Prusa, in Bithynia, was a famous physician in Rome early in the first century before Christ. He studied both rhetoric and medicine at Alexandria and at Athens. He began as a teacher of rhetoric in Rome, but, although he was the friend of Cicero, he was not very successful, and abandoned this study for the practice of medicine. He had a great deal of ability and shrewdness, but no knowledge of anatomy or physiology, and he condemned all who thought that these subjects of study were the foundation of the healing art. He specially inveighed against Hippocrates, and with some reason, for the disciples of Hippocrates had elevated the teaching of their master almost into a religion, and were bound far too closely to his authority, to the exclusion of original thought and progress.

Asclepiades had many pupils, and his teaching led to the foundation of the Medical School of the Methodists. His most important maxim was that a cure should be effected "tuto, celeriter, ac jucunde," and he believed that what the physician could do was of primary importance, and vis medicatrix natur?only secondary. He was thus directly opposed to the teaching of Hippocrates. He had little or no faith in drugs, and relied mainly upon diet, exercises and massage, and, to some extent, upon surgery. His practice of prescribing wine in liberal doses added to his popularity. It was the custom to take wine very much diluted with water, but Asclepiades ordered wine in full strength or only slightly diluted. He practised bronchotomy and tracheotomy, and recommended in suitable cases of dropsy scarification of the ankles, and advised that, in tapping, an opening as small as possible should be made. He also observed spontaneous dislocation of the hip. He was a very famous man in the Roman Republic, and was well acquainted with philosophy, especially the philosophy of the Epicureans. Although he was almost entirely ignorant of anatomy, he was far from being a quack. He had great powers of observation and natural shrewdness, and his success largely contributed to the establishment of Greek doctors and their methods in Rome. There is grim humour in his description of the Hippocratic treatise on therapeutics, which he called "a meditation on death." Pliny relates that Asclepiades wagered that he would never die of disease, and he won the wager, for he lived to old age and died of an accident!

Themison, of Laodicea, lived in the first century before Christ, and was a pupil of Asclepiades of Prusa, the founder of the School of Methodism. His views on atoms and pores led him to adopt a very simple explanation of health and disease, for he considered that these pores must be either constricted or dilated, and the aim of the physician should be to dilate the constriction, and vice versa. This epitomized system of medicine did away with the use of many classes of drugs, and, from its simplicity, was quickly learned. A jeering opponent of the system of the Methodici said that it could be taught in six months, and Galen, in later years, ridiculed it, and called its practitioners "the asses of Thessaly."

The great fault of Dogmatism was its absolute reliance on the wisdom of Hippocrates, and Methodism was marred by its insufficiency and sophistry.

In spite of his extravagant theories, Themison possessed skill in practice. He was the first physician to describe rheumatism, and he also is thought to have been the pioneer in the medicinal use of leeches. A book on elephantiasis ascribed to him is not definitely known to be authentic. It is worthy of note that he was anxious to write on hydrophobia, but a case he had seen in early youth so impressed his mind with horror that the mere thought of the disease caused him to suffer some of the symptoms.

The views of the Methodists were less extreme than those of the Dogmatists and Empirics. Celsus wrote of the Methodists: "They assert that the knowledge of no cause whatever bears the least relation to the method of cure; and that it is sufficient to observe some general symptoms of distempers; and that there are three kinds of diseases, one bound, another loose, and the third is a mixture of these."[11]

There were several physicians of the name of Themison at different times, and it is probably the founder of the Methodici who was satirized by Juvenal thus:--

"How many patients Themison dispatched In one short autumn."[12]

The joke which is based on attributing a cure to Nature alone, and death solely to the physician's want of skill, is one of the most time-honoured.

Themison lived at the close of the Roman Republic, and it will now be necessary to consider the state of the healing art in Rome under the rule of the emperors.

Julius Caesar--one of the first triumvirate--invaded and conquered Gaul and Britain, and after these great military achievements, found that he could not sheath his sword until he had met in battle his rival Pompey. Caesar defeated Pompey at Pharsalia, in Thessaly (48 B.C.), and pursued him to Egypt. Pompey was murdered in Egypt, and his last followers finally defeated in Spain, and in 45 B.C. Julius Caesar returned to Rome, and was declared perpetual imperator. On March 15, 44 B.C., he was assassinated. It is possible that the career of this great man may have promoted the surgery of the battlefield, but his reign as Emperor was too short, and the political situation of his time too acute, to permit of much progress in the arts of peace generally, and in the medical art particularly. Julius Caesar bestowed the right of Roman citizenship on all medical practitioners in the city.

Referring to the death of Julius Caesar, Suetonius writes that among so many wounds there was none that was mortal, in the opinion of the surgeon Antistus, except the second, which he received in the breast.

Octavianus was appointed one of the second triumvirate, his colleagues being Mark Antony and Lepidus. Lepidus was first forced out of the triumvirate, and Octavianus and Mark Antony then came into conflict. During these rivalries, a great civic work was accomplished by Marcus Agrippa, who built the aqueduct known as Aqua Julia. A landmark in history is the battle of Actium, in which Octavianus defeated Mark Antony and his ally Cleopatra, and within a few years Octavianus was proclaimed Emperor as Augustus Caesar (27 B.C.). Under his rule Rome greatly prospered, and we shall now consider the state of medicine and of sanitation during his illustrious reign.

In the Roman Empire there was a spirit of toleration abroad, "and the various modes of worship which prevailed in the Roman world were all considered by the people as equally true; by the philosopher, as equally false; and by the magistrate, as equally useful. And thus toleration produced not only mutual indulgence, but even religious concord" (Gibbon).

The systems of philosophy in vogue were those of the Stoics, the Platonists, the Academics, and the Epicureans, and of these only the Platonists had any belief in God, who was to them an idea rather than a Supreme Being. The great aim of both the wise and the foolish was to glorify their nationality, and their beliefs, their rites, and their superstitions, were all for the glory of mighty Rome.

Educated Romans were able to speak and write both Latin and Greek, and the latter language was the vehicle used by men of science and of letters.

The population of the city of Rome at the beginning of the Augustan age was not less than half a million of people, and probably exceeded this number. There was no middle class, a comparatively small number of gentry, a very numerous plebs or populace, and many slaves. The Emperor Augustus boasted that after the war with Sextus Pompeius he handed over 30,000 slaves, who had been serving with the enemy, to their masters to be punished. The slaves were looked upon by their masters as chattels. The plebs had the spirit of paupers and, to keep them contented and pacific, were fed and shown brutalizing spectacles in the arenas. Augustus wrote that he gave the people wild-beast hunts in the circus and amphitheatres twenty-six times, in which about 3,500 animals were killed. It was his custom to watch the Circensian games from his palace in view of a multitude of spectators.

Throughout the country generally agriculture prospered, and the supply of various grasses for feeding cattle in the winter increased the multitude of the flocks and herds; great attention was given also to mines and fisheries and all forms of industry. Virgil praised his beautiful and fertile country:--

"But no, not Medeland with its wealth of woods, Fair Ganges, Hermus thick with golden silt, Can match the praise of Italy.... Here blooms perpetual spring, and summer here In months that are not summer's; twice teem the flocks: Twice does the tree yield service of her fruit. Mark too, her cities, so many and so proud, Of mighty toil the achievement, town on town Up rugged precipices heaved and reared, And rivers gliding under ancient walls."[13]

The city of Rome was not a desirable place for medical practice, for the lower classes were degraded and thriftless, and the relatively small upper classes were tyrannical, debauched, superstitious, selfish and cruel. The younger Pliny, who was one of the best type of Romans, tried to investigate the purity of the lives of the Christians, and did not hesitate to put to torture two women, deaconesses, who belonged to the new religion, but he "could discover only an obstinate kind of superstition carried to great excess." His conduct and his opinion speak eloquently of the nature of a Roman gentleman of the Empire. As for the state of the poor under Augustus, 200,000 persons in Rome received outdoor relief. Although the rich had every luxury that desire could suggest and wealth afford, the great need of the common people was food. The city had to rely mainly on imported corn, and the price of this at times became prohibitive owing to scarcity--sometimes the result of piracy and the dangers of the sea, but often caused by artificial means owing to the merchants "cornering" the supply--and it was necessary for the State, through the Emperor, to intervene to make regulations and to distribute the grain free or below its market value. It has been computed that about 50,000 strangers lived in Rome, many of whom were adventurers.

The imperial city was the happy hunting-ground of quacks, who gave themselves high-sounding names and wore gorgeous raiment. They went about followed by a retinue of pupils and grateful patients. In some cases the patients were compelled to promise, in the event of being cured, that they would serve their doctor ever afterwards. The retinue of students, no doubt, was rather disturbing to a nervous patient, and Martial wrote:--

"Faint was I only, Symmachus, till thou Backed by an hundred students, throng'dst my bed; An hundred icy fingers chilled my brow: I had no fever; now I'm nearly dead."[14]

Besides quack doctors there were drug sellers (pharmacopola), who sold their medicines in booths or hawked them in the city and the country. In the time of the Empire the medicines of the regular practitioners were sold with a label which specified the name of the drug and of the inventor, the ingredients, the disease it was to be used for, and the method of taking it. Drug sellers dispensed cosmetics as well as medicines, and some of the itinerant dealers sold poison. The regular physicians bought medicines already compounded by the druggists, and the latter, as in our own day, prescribed as well as the physicians.

Depilatories were much in vogue, and were usually made of arsenic and unslaked lime, but also from the roots and juices of plants. They were first used only by women, but in later times also by effeminate men. Tweezers have been discovered which were adapted for pulling out hairs, and most of the depilatories were recommended to be applied after the use of the tweezers. The duty of pulling out hairs was performed by slaves.

Most of the medical practitioners in the time of Augustus were either slaves or freedmen. Posts of responsibility and of honour were sometimes assigned to freedmen, as is shown by the appointment by Nero of Helius, a freedman, to the administration of Rome in the absence of his imperial master. Cicero wrote letters to his freedman Tiro in terms of friendship and affection. The master of a great household selected a slave for his ability and aptitude, and had him trained to be the medical adviser of the household; and the skill shown by the doctor sometimes gained for him his freedom.

There were 400 slaves in one great household of Rome, and they were all executed for not having prevented the murder of their master.[15] It is recorded that physicians were sometimes compelled to do the disgusting work of mutilating slaves.[16] The price of a slave physician was fixed at sixty solidi.[17] The great majority of physicians in Rome were freedmen who had booths in which they prescribed and compounded, and they were aided by freedmen and slaves who were both assistants and pupils. The medical profession, as has been shown, never attained the same dignity as in Greece. It should be understood that there was a class of practising physicians in Rome quite distinct from the slave doctors. The following account of Lucius Horatillavus, a Roman quack of the time of Augustus, is taken from the British Medical Journal of June 10, 1911, and originated in an article in the Society Nouvelle, written by M. Fernand Mazade:--

"He was a handsome man, and came from Naples to Rome, his sole outfit being a toga made of a piece of cloth adorned with obscene pictures and a small Asiatic mitre. Like many of his kind at that day, he sold poisons and invented five or six new remedies which were more or less haphazard mixtures of wine and poisonous substances. He had the good luck to cure his first patient, Titus Cnoeus Leno, who, being a poet, straightway constituted himself the vates sacer of his physician, and induced some of his fashionable mistresses to place themselves under his hands. So profitable was Horatillavus's practice that he is said to have saved 150,000 sesterces in a few months. But for a moment his good fortune seemed to abandon him. A Roman lady, Sulpicia Pallas, died suddenly under his ministrations. This may have been due to his ignorance or carelessness; but he was accused of having poisoned his patient. This event might have been expected to bring his career to an end; but it was not long before he recovered the confidence of the people whom he deluded with his mystical language and promises of cure. He had three methods of treatment, all consisting of baths--hot, tepid, or cold-- preceded or followed by the taking of wonder-working medicines. Horatillavus treated every kind of disease, internal and external; he even practised midwifery, which was then in the hands of women. Ten years after he settled in Rome he had accumulated a fortune of some 6,000,000 sesterces. He had a villa at Tusculum, whither he went three times a month; there he led a luxurious life in the most beautiful surroundings, and there his evil fate overtook him. His orchard was his especial pride. One day he found that birds had played havoc with his figs, the like of which were not to be found in Italy. Determined to prevent similar depredations in future, he poisoned the fig trees. Continuing his walk, he plucked fruits of various kinds here and there. While eating the fruit he had culled and drinking choice wine, he put into his mouth a poisoned fig, which he had inadvertently gathered, and quickly died in convulsions. Before passing away, however, he is said to have composed his own epitaph. This M. Mazade believes he has found. It reads: "The manes of Sulpicia Pallas have avenged her. Here lies Lucius Horatillavus, physician, who poisoned himself." If the epitaph is genuine, it is a confession of guilt. The death of the quack by his own poison is a curious Nemesis. The manner of his death proves that it was accidental, as few quacks are bold enough to take their own medicines."

FOOTNOTES:

[11] "De Medic.," lib. 1.

[12] "Sat.," x, 221.

[13] Rhodes's version.

[14] Handerson's translation.

[15] "Tacit. Annal.," xiv, 43.

[16] "Paulus," vol. ii, p. 379.

[17] "Just. Cod.," vii.

CHAPTER VI.

IN THE REIGN OF THE CAESARS--TO THE DEATH OF NERO.

Augustus--His illnesses--Antonius Musa--Menenas--Tiberius-- Caligula--

Claudius--Nero--Seneca--Astrology--Archiater--Women poisoners--Oculists in Rome.

Long before the settlement of the constitutional status of Augustus in 27 B.C., he had undertaken many reforms. In 34 B.C., Agrippa, under the influence of Augustus, had improved the water supply of Rome by restoring the Aqua Marcia, and Augustus had repaired and enlarged the cloac? and repaired the principal streets. Road commissions were appointed 27 B.C. The Aqua Virgo was built 19 B.C. Many of the collegia, or guilds, founded for the promotion of the interests of professions and trades had been misused for political purposes, and Augustus deprived many of them of their charters. Cur? or commissions, were appointed to superintend public works, streets and the water-supply; and the Tiber was dredged, cleansed and widened, and its liability to overflow reduced. No new building could be built more than 70 ft. high. Augustus also established fire brigades. It has been said that he found the city built of brick and left it built of marble.

He revived many old religious customs, such as the Augury of Public Health, and identified himself closely with the rites and customs of the people. He inculcated that sense of duty which the Romans called pietas, and attempted to improve the morals of the citizens by the enactment of sumptuary laws; the philosophers hoped to do good in the same direction by appealing to the intellect and reason, a method that was equally ineffectual. Marriages and an increased birth-rate were encouraged, and parents were honoured and given special privileges. The wisdom and prudence of Augustus were strangely accompanied by credulity and superstition. He was a profound believer in omens, and attached great importance to astrology. His horoscope showed that he was born under the sign of Capricorn.

He suffered from various illnesses, although in his younger days he looked handsome and athletic. He carefully nursed his health against his many infirmities, avoiding chiefly the free use of the bath; but he was often rubbed with oil, and sweated in a stove, after which he was bathed in tepid water, warmed either by a fire, or by being exposed to the heat of the sun. When, on account of his nerves, he was obliged to have recourse to sea-water, or the waters of Albula, he was contented with sitting over a wooden tub, (which he called by a Spanish name, Dureta), and plunging his hands and feet in the water by turns.[18] His physician was Antonius Musa, to whom was erected, by public subscription, a statue near that of Aculapius. During an attack of congestion of the liver when heat failed to give relief, Antonius Musa advised cold applications for the Emperor, which had the desired effect. Suetonius, the historian, wrote that this was "a desperate and doubtful method of cure." A more desperate and doubtful method of cure, however, was carried out by the same physician. He successfully banished an attack of sciatica that greatly troubled Augustus by the expedient of beating the affected part with a stick. Antonius Musa received honours from Augustus, and the Emperor also exempted all physicians from the payment of taxes, and from other public obligations.

In the time of Augustus natural philosophy made little progress, and Virgil strongly desired its advancement. Human anatomy, as a study, had not been introduced, and physiology was almost unknown. In medicine, the standard of practice was the writings of Hippocrates, and the Materia Medica consisted of remedies suggested by the whimsical notions of their inventors.

Pliny wrote that the water cure was the principal remedy in his day, as it was indeed throughout the Empire, and it was certainly the most popular. Seneca was very severe on the sentiment of a poem written by Menenas, the friend and counsellor of Augustus, but it serves to reveal some of the most dreaded maladies of the time:--

"Though racked with gout in hand and foot, Though cancer deep should strike its root, Though palsy shake my feeble thighs, Though hideous lump on shoulder rise, From flaccid gum teeth drop away; Yet all is well if life but stay."

Malaria was one of the principal causes of mortality in and near Rome in the reign of Augustus Caesar.

Augustus's fatal illness occurred in A.D. 14 from chronic diarrhoea, and the Emperor, like the true Roman that he was, displayed great calmness and fortitude in his last days.

Tiberius succeeded to the throne in A.D. 14, and began a career of infamy. How little knowledge was likely to gain from his patronage is shown by the fact, recorded by Pliny, that the shop and tools of the artist who discovered how to make glass malleable were destroyed. Assassins and perpetrators of every abomination were the fit companions of this tyrant.

Thrasyllus, the astrologer, lived with Tiberius, who was a firm believer in the magic arts. This reign is made illustrious in the history of medicine by the work of Celsus.

Caligula, who became Emperor in A.D. 34, was guilty of the most inhuman conduct. Criminals were given to the wild beasts for their food, and even people of honourable rank had their faces branded with hot irons as a punishment by order of this mad tyrant.

Claudius, the successor of Caligula, completed some very important public works in his reign, including great aqueducts and drains, but learning was at a low ebb in his day. Claudius Etruscus, the freedman of the Emperor Claudius, erected baths referred to by Martial. The ruins of the arches of the Aqua Claudia still remain.

Thrasyllus, a son of the astrologer who lived in the time of Tiberius, is said to have predicted to Nero the dignity of the purple. Nero would have been favourably disposed towards physicians if he had heeded the advice of his tutor, Seneca, who wrote: "People pay the doctor for his trouble; for his kindness they still remain in his debt." "Great reverence and love is due to both the teacher and the doctor. We have received from them priceless benefits; from the doctor, health and life; from the teacher, the noble culture of the soul. Both are our friends, and deserve our most sincere thanks, not so much by their merchantable art, as by their frank goodwill."[19] The practice of necromancy in the time of Nero had grown to such an extent that an edict of banishment was issued against all magicians, but this did not lessen the popularity of the magicians, who indeed prospered under the semblance of persecution, and were honoured in times of public difficulty and danger. The practice of astrology came from the Chaldeans, and was introduced into Greece in the third century before Christ. It was accepted by all classes, but specially by the Stoic philosophers. In 319 B.C., Cornelius Hispallus banished the Chaldeans from Rome, and ordered them to leave Italy within ten days. In 33 B.C., they were again banished by Marcus Agrippa, and Augustus also issued an edict against them. They were punished sometimes by death, and their calling must have been lucrative to induce them to continue in spite of the severe punishments to which they made themselves liable. The penal laws against them, however, were in operation only intermittently. They were consulted by all classes, from the Emperor downwards.

There were many physicians in the reign of Nero, but none of great eminence. Andromachus was physician to the Emperor, and had the title of archiater, which means "chief of the physicians."

An account of the archiaters is of interest. The name was applied to Christ by St. Jerome. There were two classes of archiaters in time, the one class called archiatri sancti palati; the other, archiatri populares. The former attended the Emperor, and were court physicians; the latter attended the people. Although Nero appointed the first archiater, the name is not commonly used in Latin until the time of Constantine, and the division into two classes probably dates from about that time. The archiatri sancti palati were of high rank, and were the judges of disputes between physicians. The Archiatri had many privileges conferred upon them. They, and their wives and children, did not have to pay taxes. They were not obliged to give lodgings to soldiers in the provinces, and they could not be put in prison. These privileges applied more especially to the higher class. When an archiater sancti palati ceased attendance on the Emperor he took the title of ex-archiater. The title comes archiatorum means "count of the Archiatri," and gave rank among the high nobility of the Empire.

The archiatri populares attended the sick poor, and each city had five, seven or ten, according to its size. Rome had fourteen of these officers, besides one for the vestal virgins, and one for the gymnasia. They were paid by the Government for attending the poor, but were not restricted to this class of practice, and were well paid by their prosperous patients. Their office was more lucrative but not so honourable as that of the archiaters of the palace. The archiatri populares were elected by the people themselves.

Suetonius describes the treatment Nero underwent for the improvement of his voice: "He would lie upon his back with a sheet of lead upon his breast, clear his stomach and bowels by vomits and clysters, and forbear the eating of fruits, or food prejudicial to his voice." He built, at great expense, magnificent public baths supplied from the sea and from hot springs, and was the first to build a public gymnasium in Rome.

There is reason to believe that in the time of Nero there was a class of women poisoners. Nero employed one of these women, Locusta by name, and after she had poisoned Britannicus, rewarded her with a great estate in land, and placed disciples with her to be instructed in her nefarious trade.

There was also a very ignorant class of oculists in Rome in the time of Nero, but at Marseilles Demosthenes Philalethes was deservedly celebrated, and his book on diseases of the eye was in use for several centuries. The eye doctors of Rome employed ointments almost entirely, and about two hundred seals have been discovered which had been attached to pots of eye salves, each seal bearing the inventor's and proprietor's name. In the time of Galen, these quack oculists were very numerous, and Galen inveighs against them. Martial satirized them: "Now you are a gladiator who once were an ophthalmist; you did as a doctor what you do as a gladiator." "The blear-eyed Hylas would have paid you sixpence, O Quintus; one eye is gone, he will still pay threepence; make haste and take it, brief is your chance; when he is blind, he will pay you nothing." The oculists of Alexandria were very proficient, and some of their followers, at various times throughout the period of the Roman Empire, were remarkably skilful. Their literature has perished, but it is believed that they were able to operate on cataract.

With the death of Nero in A.D. 68, the direct line of the Caesars became extinct.

FOOTNOTES:

[18] Suetonius: "Lives of the Caesars," lxxxii.

[19] Seneca "De Benefic.," vi.

CHAPTER VII.

PHYSICIANS FROM THE TIME OF AUGUSTUS TO THE DEATH OF NERO.

Celsus--His life and works--His influence on Medicine--Meges of Sidon--Apollonius of Tyana--Alleged miracles--Vettius Valleus--Scribonius Longus--Andromachus--Thessalus of Tralles--Pliny.

Aulus Cornelius Celsus lived in the reigns of Augustus and Tiberius. References in his works show that he either lived at the same time as Themison or shortly after him. Verona has been claimed as his birthplace, but the purity of his literary style shows that he lived for a considerable time in Rome, and he was probably educated there. In Pliny's account of the history of medicine, Celsus is not mentioned as having practised in Rome, and it is almost certain that he combined the practice of medicine with the study of science and literary pursuits; his practice was not general, but restricted to his friends and dependents. His writings show that he had a clinical knowledge of disease and a considerable amount of medical experience. He wrote not only on medicine but also on history, philosophy, jurisprudence and rhetoric, agriculture and military tactics. His great medical work, "De Medicina," comprises eight books. He properly begins with the history of medicine, and then proceeds to discuss the merits of the controversy between the Dogmatici and the Empirici. The first two books deal with general principles and with diet, and the remaining books with particular diseases; the third and fourth with internal diseases, the fifth and sixth with external diseases and pharmacy, and the last two are surgical, and of great merit and importance. In his methods of treatment there can be discerned the influence of Asclepiades of Prusa, and the Hippocratic principle of aiding rather than opposing nature, but some of his work displays originality. His devotion to Hippocrates hindered very much the exercise of his own powers, and set a bad example, in this respect, to his successors.

He was rather free in the use of the lancet, but not to the same extent as his contemporaries, and he advocated the use of free purgation as well as bleeding. He never could rid his mind of the orthodox humoral theories of his predecessors.

(1) Surgery.--Although Celsus is the first writer in Rome to deal fully with surgical procedures, it must not be inferred that the practice of this art began to be developed in his time, for surgery was then much more advanced than medicine. Many major operations were performed, and it is very instructive for doctors of the present day to learn that much that is considered modern was well understood by the ancients. There is no greater fallacy than to suppose that medical practice generally, and surgery in particular, has reached no eminence except in very recent times. The operation of crushing a stone in the bladder was devised at Alexandria by Ammonius Lithotomos, (287 B.C.), and is thus described by Celsus:--

"A hook or crotchet is fixed upon the stone in such a way as easily to hold it firm, even when shaken, so that it may not revolve backward; then an iron instrument is used, of moderate thickness, thin at the front end but blunt, which, when applied to the stone and struck at the other end, cleaves it. Great care must be taken that the instrument do not come into contact with the bladder itself, and that nothing fall upon it by the breaking of the stone."

Celsus describes plastic operations for the repair of the nose, lips and ears, though these operations are generally supposed to have been recently devised.

He describes lithotomy, and operations upon the eye, as practised at Alexandria, both probably introduced there from India. Subcutaneous urethrotomy was also practised in his time.

Trephining had long been a well-known operation of surgery. There is an account in detail of how amputation should be performed.

The teaching of Celsus in reference to dislocations and fractures is remarkably advanced. Dislocations, he points out, should be reduced before inflammation sets in, and in failure of union of fractures, he recommends extension and the rubbing together of the ends of the broken bone to promote union. If necessary, after minor measures have failed to promote union, he recommends an incision down to the ends of the bones, and the open incision and the fracture will heal at the same time.

It is interesting to find that Celsus knew of the danger of giving purgatives in strangulated rupture of the bowels. For uncomplicated rupture he recommends reduction by taxis and operation. Cauterization of the canal is part of the operation. He also gives careful directions for removing foreign bodies from the ears.

Celsus writes very fully on hemorrhage, and describes the method of tying two ligatures upon a blood-vessel, and severing it between the ligatures. His method of amputating in cases of gangrene by a simple circular incision was in use down to comparatively modern times. He describes catheterization, plastic operations on the face, the resection of ribs for the cure of sinuses in the chest walls, operation for cataract, ear disease curable by the use of the syringe, and operations for goitre. These goitre operations are generally supposed to be a recent triumph of surgery.

Celsus also had knowledge of dentistry, for he writes of teeth extraction by means of forceps, the fastening of loose teeth with gold wire, and a method of bursting decayed and hollow teeth by means of peppercorns forced into the cavity. He has described also many of the most difficult operations in obstetrics.

When it is remembered that Celsus lived centuries before the introduction of chloroform and ether, it is wonderful to contemplate what was accomplished long ago.

The qualities which should distinguish a surgeon were described by Celsus thus: "He should not be old, his hand should be firm and steady, and he should be able to use his left hand equally with his right; his sight should be clear, and his mind calm and courageous, so that he need not hurry during an operation and cut less than required, as if the screams of the patient made no impression upon him."

(2) Anatomy.--Celsus understood fairly well the situation of the internal organs, and knew well the anatomy of the chest and female pelvis. His knowledge of the skeleton was particularly complete and accurate. He describes very fully the bones of the head, including the perforated plate of the ethmoid bone, the sutures, the teeth, and the skeletal bones generally. Portal states that Celsus knew of the semicircular canals. He understood the structure of the joints, and points out that cartilage is part of their formation.

Celsus wrote: "It is both cruel and superfluous to dissect the bodies of the living, but to dissect those of the dead is necessary for learners, for they ought to know the position and order which dead bodies show better than a living and wounded man. But even the other things which can only be observed in the living, practice itself will show in the cures of the wounded, a little more slowly but somewhat more tenderly."

(3) Medicine.--His treatment of fevers was excellent, for he recognized that fever was an effort of Nature to throw off morbid materials. His recipes are

not so complicated, but more sensible and effective than those of his immediate successors. He understood the use of enemas and artificial feeding. In cases of insanity he recognized that improvement followed the use of narcotics in the treatment of the accompanying insomnia. He recognized also morbid illusions. He recommended lotions and salves for the treatment of some eye diseases.

Although Celsus practised phlebotomy, he discountenanced very strongly its excessive use. The physicians in Rome, in his time, carried bleeding to great extremes. "It is not," wrote Celsus, "a new thing to let blood from the veins, but it is new that there is scarcely a malady in which blood is not drawn. Formerly they bled young men, and women who were not pregnant, but it had not been seen till our days that children, pregnant women, and old men were bled." The reason for bleeding the strong and plethoric was to afford outlet to an excessive supply of blood, and the weak were similarly treated to get rid of evil humours, so that hardly any sick person could escape this drastic treatment.

Emetics were greatly used in the time of Celsus. Voluptuaries made use of them to excite an appetite for food, and they used them after eating heavy meals to prepare the stomach for a second bout of gluttony. Many gourmands took an emetic daily. Celsus said that emetics should not be used as a frequent practice if the attainment of old age was desired.

Celsus excelled as a compiler, and had the faculty of selecting the most admirable contributions to the art of healing from previous medical writers. His writings also give an account of what was best in the medical practice of Rome about his own time. He had a great love for learning, and it is remarkable that he was attracted to the study of medicine, for he was a patrician, and members of his class considered study of that kind beneath the dignity of their rank.

In the Augustan age, when literature in Rome reached its highest level, the literary style of Celsus was fit to be classed with that of the great writers of his time. He was never quoted as a great authority on medicine or surgery by later medical writers; and Pliny refers to him as a literary man, and not as a practising physician. From the fact that he elaborated no new system, and founded no new medical sect, it is not strange that he had no disciples.

In later centuries his works were used as a textbook for students, not only for the information they supplied, but also because of their excellence as literature.

Parts of the foregoing synopsis of the writings of Celsus are drawn from the writings of Hermann Baas and of Berdoe.

Meges of Sidon (20 B.C.) was a famous surgeon who practised in Rome shortly before the time of Celsus. He was regarded by Celsus as the most skilful surgeon of that period, and his works, of which nothing now remains, were quoted by Celsus, and also referred to by Pliny. Meges was a follower of Themison. He is said to have invented instruments used in cutting for stone, and he wrote on tumours of the breast and dislocation of the knee. There have been several famous doctors called Eudemus. One of these was an anatomist in the third century before Christ, and a contemporary, according to Galen, of Herophilus and Erasistratus. He gave great attention to the anatomy and physiology of the nervous system. There was, however, another Eudemus, a physician of Rome, who became entangled in an intrigue with the wife of the son of the Emperor Tiberius. He aided her in an attempt to poison her husband in A.D. 23. He was put to torture, and finally executed by order of Tiberius.

Apollonius of Tyana was born four years before the Christian era, in the time of Augustus Caesar, and is known chiefly for the parallel that has been drawn by ancient and modern writers between his supposed miracles and those of the Saviour. His doings as described by Philostratus are extraordinary and incredible, and he was put forward by the Eclectics in opposition to the unique powers claimed by Christ and believed in by His followers. Apollonius is said to have studied the philosophy of the Platonic, Sceptic, Epicurean,

Peripatetic and Pythagorean schools, and to have adopted that of Pythagoras. He schooled himself in early manhood in the asceticism of that philosophy. He abstained from animal food and strong drink, wore white linen garments and sandals made of bark, and let his hair grow long. For five years he preserved a mystic silence, and during this period the truths of philosophy became known to him. He had interviews with the Magi in Asia Minor, and learned strange secrets from the Brahmans in India. In Greece he visited the temples and oracles, and exercised his powers of healing. Like Pythagoras, he travelled far and wide, disputing about philosophy wherever he went, and he gained an extraordinary reputation for magical powers. The priests of the temples gave him divine honours and sent the sick to him to be cured. He arrived in Rome just after an edict had been promulgated by Nero against magicians. He was tried before Telesinus, the consul, and Tigellinus, the base favourite of the Emperor. He was acquitted by Telesinus because of his love of philosophy, and by Tigellinus because of his fear of magic. Subsequently, at Alexandria, Apollonius, in virtue of his magic power, affirmed that he would make Vespasian emperor, and afterwards became the friend of Titus, Vespasian's son. On the accession of Domitian, Apollonius stirred up the provinces against him, and was ordered to be brought in custody to Rome, but he surrendered himself to the authorities, and was brought into the presence of the Emperor to be questioned. He began to praise Nerva, and was immediately ordered to prison and to chains. It is said that he miraculously escaped, and spent the remainder of his days in Ephesus.

The relation of Apollonius to the art of medicine is connected with his visits, on his travels, to the temples of Aculapius, and his healing of the sick and alleged triumph over the laws of Nature. He was also credited with raising the dead, casting out devils and other miracle-working that appears to have been borrowed from the life of Christ. No doubt he was a genuine philosopher and follower of Pythagoras. His history is, on the whole, worthy of belief, except the part relating to miracles. It is noteworthy that he did not claim for himself miraculous power. Newman in his "Life of Apollonius" takes the view that the account of the miracles of Apollonius is derived from the narrative of Christ's miracles, and has been concocted by people anxious to degrade the character of the Saviour. The attempt to make him appear as a pagan Christ has been renewed in recent years.

In the realm of medical practice he succeeded by imposture probably, but also in a genuine way by means of suggestion, and no doubt he had also acquired medical knowledge from study and travelling among people who had healing powers and items of medical knowledge perhaps unknown at the present day.

Vettius (or Vectius) Valleus, was of equestrian rank but he did not confer any honour on the medical profession. He was one of the lewd companions of Messalina, the wife of the Emperor Claudius, and was put to death in A.D. 48. He was a believer in Themison's doctrines, and is said by Pliny[20] to have founded a new medical sect, but nearly all the Methodici attempted to create a new sect by adding to, or subtracting a little from, the tenets of Methodism.

Scribonius Largus (about A.D. 45) was physician to Claudius and accompanied him to Britain. He wrote several medical books, and is reputed to have used electricity for the relief of headaches.

Andromachus, the elder, was physician to Nero, and the first archiater. He was born in Crete. He was the inventor of a compound medicine called after himself, "Theriaca Andromachi." He gave directions for making it in a poem of 174 lines. This poem is quoted by Galen, who explains that Andromachus gave his instructions a poetical form to assist memory, and to prevent the likelihood of alteration.

Andromachus, the younger, was the son of the first archiater, and was, like his father, physician to Nero. He wrote a book on Pharmacy, in three volumes.

Thessalus of Tralles, in Lydia, lived in Rome in the reign of Nero, and dedicated one of his books to the Emperor. He was a charlatan with no medical knowledge, but with a good deal of ability and assurance. He said that medicine surpassed all other arts, and he surpassed all other physicians.

His father had been a weaver, and in his youth Thessalus followed the same calling, and never had any medical training. This did not prevent him, however, from acquiring a great reputation as a doctor, and making a fortune from medical practice. At first, he associated himself with the views of the Methodici, but afterwards amended them as he thought fit, until he had convinced the public, and perhaps also himself, that he was the founder of a new and true system of medicine. He spoke in very disrespectful and violent terms of his predecessors, and said that no man before him had done anything to advance the science of medicine. Besides having an endowment of natural shrewdness and ability, he was equipped with great powers of self-advertisement, and could cajole the rich and influential. He was an adept in the art of flattery. Galen often refers to him, and always with contempt. Thessalus was able, so he said, to teach the medical art in six months, and he surrounded himself with a retinue of artisans, weavers, cooks, butchers, and so on, who were allowed to kill or cure his patients. Sprengel states that, after the time of Thessalus, the doctors of Rome forbore to take their pupils with them on professional visits.

He began a method of treatment for chronic and obstinate cases. The first three days of the treatment were given up to the use of vegetable drugs, emetics, and strict dietary. Then followed fasting, and finally a course of tonics and restoratives. He is said to have used colchicum for gout. The tomb of Thessalus on the Appian Way was to be seen in Pliny's time. It bore the arrogant device "Conqueror of Physicians." The success of Thessalus seems a proof of the cynical belief that the public take a man's worth at his own estimate.

Pliny, the elder, lived from A.D. 23 to 79, dying during the eruption of Vesuvius when Pompeii and Herculaneum were destroyed. He was not a scientific man, but was a prodigious recorder of information on all subjects. Much of this information is inaccurate, for he was not able to discriminate between the true and the false, or to assign to facts their relative value.

His great book on Natural History includes many subjects that cannot properly be considered as belonging to Natural History. It consists of thirty-six books and an index, and the author stated that the work dealt with twenty thousand important matters, and was compiled from two thousand volumes.

Although Pliny was not a physician he writes about medicine, and paints a picture of the state of medical knowledge of his time. His own opinions on the subject are of no value. He believed that magic is a branch of medicine, and was optimistic enough to hold that there is a score of remedies for every disease. His writings upon the virtues of medicines derived from the human body, from fish, and from plants are more picturesque than accurate.

FOOTNOTES:

[20] H. N., xxix, 5.

CHAPTER VIII.

THE FIRST AND SECOND CENTURIES OF THE CHRISTIAN ERA.

Athens--Pneumatism--Eclectics--Agathinus--Aretemes--Archigenes--
Dioscorides--Cassius Felix--Pestilence in Rome--Ancient surgical instruments--
Herodotus--Heliodorus--Caius Aurelianus--Soranus-- Rufus of Ephesus--
Marinus--Quintus.

Athens, of Cilicia, a Stoic and Peripatetic, founded in Rome the sect of the Pneumatists about the year A.D. 69. It was inspired by the philosophy of Plato. The pneuma, or spirit, was in their opinion the cause of health and of disease. They believed that dilatation of the arteries drives onward the pneuma, and contraction of the arteries drives it in a contrary direction. The pneuma passes from the heart to the arteries. Their theories also had reference to the elements. Thus, the union of heat and moisture maintains health; heat and dryness cause acute diseases; cold and moisture cause chronic diseases; cold and dryness cause mental depression, and at death there are both dryness and coldness. In spite of these strange opinions the Pneumatists made some scientific progress, and recognized some diseases hitherto unknown. Galen wrote of the Pneumatists: "They would rather betray their country than abjure their opinions." The founder of the sect of Pneumatists was a very prolific writer, for the twenty-ninth volume of one of his works is quoted by Oribasius. The teaching of the Pneumatists speedily gave way to that of the Eclectics, of whom Galen was by far the most celebrated. They tried to reconcile the teaching of the Dogmatists, Methodists, and Empirics, and adopted what they considered to be the best teaching of each sect. The Eclectics were very similar to, if not identical with, the Episynthetics, founded by a pupil of Athens, by name, Agathinus. He was a Spartan by birth. He is frequently quoted by Galen, but none of his writings are extant.

Aretemes, the Cappadocian, practised in Rome in the first century of our era, in the reign of Nero or Vespasian. He published a book on medicine, still extant, which displays a great knowledge of the symptoms of disease very accurately described, and reliable for purposes of diagnosis. He was the first to reveal the glandular nature of the kidneys, and for the first time employed cantharides as a counter-irritant (Portal, vol. i, p. 62). It is not surprising that Aretemes followed rather closely the teaching of Hippocrates, but he considered it right to check some of "the natural actions" of the body, which Hippocrates thought were necessary for the restoration of health. He was not against phlebotomy, and used strong purgatives and also narcotics. He was less tied to the opinions of any sect than the physicians of his time, and was both wonderfully accurate in his opinions and reliable in treatment. Aretemes condemned the operation of tracheotomy first proposed by Asclepiades, and held "that the heat of the inflammation becomes greater from the wound and contributes to the suffocation, and the patient coughs; and even if he escapes this danger, the lips of the wound do not unite, for both are cartilaginous and unable to grow together." He believed, also, that elephantiasis was contagious. The writings of Aretemes consist of eight books, and there have been many editions in various languages. Only a few chapters are missing.

Archigenes was a pupil of Agathinus, and is mentioned by Juvenal. He was born in Syria and practised in Rome in the reign of Trajan, A.D. 98-117. He introduced new and very obscure terms into his writings. He wrote on the pulse, and on this Galen wrote a commentary. He also proposed a classification of fevers, but his views on this subject were speculative theories, and not based upon practical experience and observation. To him is due the credit of suggesting opium for the treatment of dysentery, and he also described accurately the symptoms and progress of abscess of the liver. By some authorities he is thought to have belonged to the sect of the Pneumatici.

Dioscorides was the author of a famous treatise on Materia Medica. At different times there were several physicians of this name. He lived shortly after Pliny in the first century, but there is some doubt as to the exact time. His five books were the standard work on Materia Medica for many centuries after his death. He compiled an account of all the materials in use medicinally, and gave a description of their properties and action. This entailed great knowledge and industry, and is of value as showing what drugs were used in his time. Since then practically the whole of Materia Medica has been changed. He held largely to the orthodox beliefs of Dogmatism, but a great deal of what he recommends is not comprised in the doctrines of this sect, and is decidedly Empirical. It is difficult or impossible to identify many of the drugs referred to by Dioscorides, partly because his descriptions are brief, partly because the mistakes of his predecessors are found in his book.

He exercised as much authority in Materia Medica as Galen did in the practice of medicine, and the successors of each were content, in the main, to follow blindly. A large work was published in England in 1806 to illustrate the plants of Greece described in the treatises of Dioscorides.

Cassius Felix is supposed to have lived in the first century of our era, but practically nothing is known of his history. He wrote a book on medicine consisting of eighty-four questions on medical and physical subjects and the answers to them.

In A.D. 79, after the eruption of Vesuvius, there was a great pestilence in Rome, which historians ascribed to the pollution of the air by the eruption. Fugitives crowded into Rome from the devastated part of the country, and there was great poverty and an accumulation of filth in the city, which was, doubtless, the true cause of the pestilence. Treatment of fever at that time was very imperfect at the best, and proper means of prevention and treatment were entirely absent in time of pestilence. It has been computed that ten thousand people died daily at that time in Rome and the surrounding district. Excavations at Pompeii have done a great deal to reveal the state of surgical knowledge towards the end of the first century of our era. Professor Vulpes has written an account of the surgical instruments recovered from the ruins, and there is a collection of ancient surgical instruments in the Naples museum. Vaginal and rectal specula have been found: also a forceps for removing fractured pieces of bone from the surface of the brain. There is an instrument considered by Professor Vulpes to have been used as an artery forceps. Other instruments discovered are: Forceps for removing tumours; instruments for tapping in cases of dropsy (such an instrument was described by Celsus); seven varieties of probes; bronze catheters; 89 specimens of pincers; various kinds of knives, bone-elevators, lancets, spatulas, cauteries, saws, and trephines.[21]

There were several physicians and surgeons of the name of Herodotus. A famous surgeon of that name lived in Rome about A.D. 100. He was a pupil of Athens, and is quoted by Galen and Oribasius. This Herodotus, according to Baas, was the discoverer of pomegranate root as a remedy for tapeworm.

Heliodorus was a famous surgeon of Rome, and lived about the same time as Herodotus. He was the contemporary of Juvenal. He performed internal urethrotomy, and wrote on amputations, injuries of the head, and hernia.

Caius Aurelianus probably lived in the first century of the Christian era, but some writers believe that he was a contemporary of Galen and a rival, because the one never mentions nor is mentioned by the other; but this view is unnecessarily severe upon the standard of medical ethics attained by the leaders of the profession in early times. From the style of his writings, it has been deduced that Caius Aurelianus was not a native of Greece or of Rome. He belonged strictly to the sect of the Methodici, and his writings are important as revealing very fully the teaching of this sect. He mentions some diseases not previously described, and had a good knowledge of symptoms. He divided diseases into two classes, acute and chronic, or, more in conformity with the terminology of the Methodici, those of constriction and those of relaxation. Aurelianus did not concern himself with inquiring into the causation of diseases. His method was to find out the class to which a disease belonged, and to treat it accordingly. He was very practical in his views, and did a great deal to place treatment upon a satisfactory basis. His chief weakness was his failure to recognize the various differences and gradations, and he attached far too much importance to the two classes recognized by his school. He withheld active treatment until he had ascertained to his own satisfaction the class to which the disease belonged. Caius Aurelianus wrote three books on acute diseases and five on chronic diseases. He cites the case of a patient who was cured of dropsy by tapping, and of a person who was shot through the lungs with an arrow and recovered. He agreed with Aretemes in condemning tracheotomy. His books are not written in a good literary style.

Soranus, of Ephesus, was an eminent physician of the Methodist school, who practised in Rome in the reigns of Trajan and Hadrian. He wrote a great work on diseases of women, of which a Greek manuscript, copied in the fifteenth century, was discovered in La Bibliotheque Royale in Paris by Dietz, who was commissioned by the Prussian Government to explore the public libraries of Europe. The same investigator also discovered another copy of the work, in a worse state of preservation however, in the Vatican library. Parts of the writings of Soranus are preserved in the writings of Oribasius. There is no doubt that Soranus was a very accomplished obstetrician and gynecologist. His description of the uterus and its ligaments and the displacements to which the organ is liable reveals a practical knowledge of anatomy. Unlike most medical writers of ancient times, he did not adopt the method of recording various methods of treatment copied from previous writers, but his textbook is systematic. In writing about a disease he begins with a historical introduction, and proceeds to describe its causation, symptoms, and course, and the treatment of its various phases. His account of obstetrics shows that the art was well understood in his time. His work on the subjects of dystocia, inflammation of the uterus, and prolapse is perhaps the best. He refers also to hysterectomy. It is interesting to note that he used the speculum. He describes the qualifications of a good midwife. She need not know very much anatomy, but should have been trained in dietetics, materia medica, and minor surgical manipulations, such as version. She should be free from all corrupt and criminal practices, temperate, and not superstitious or avaricious.

In dealing with the subject of inversion of the uterus, Soranus points out that this condition may be caused by traction on the cord. It is noteworthy that he recognized the method of embryotomy as necessary when other measures had failed.

In his time leprosy was very prevalent. It had probably been brought in the first place from the East into Italy by Pompey. Some of the remedies used by Soranus for this disease are to be found in the works of Galen. Soranus wrote books on other medical subjects, but there is difficulty in deciding as to what is spurious and what is genuine in the works attributed to his authorship. There were other physicians of the same name. Galen quotes a book by Soranus on pharmacy, and C鎁ius Aurelianus one on fevers. He is also quoted by Tertullian, and by Paulus Aineta, who writes that Soranus was one of the first Greek physicians to describe the guinea-worm. Soranus, in the opinion of St. Augustine, was Medicin?auctor nobilissimus. He was far removed from the prejudices and superstitions of his time, as is shown by his denunciation of magical incantations.

Rufus, of Ephesus, also lived in the reign of Trajan (A.D. 98-117). His books reveal the state of anatomical knowledge at Alexandria before the time of Galen. The recurrent nerves were then recently discovered. He considered the spleen a useless organ. He understood that pressure on the nerves and not on the carotid arteries causes loss of voice, and that the nerves proceed from the brain, and are sensory and motor. The heart, he considered, was the seat of life, and he observed that its left ventricle is smaller and thicker than the right. The method of checking bleeding from blood-vessels by torsion was known to him. He demonstrated the investing membrane of the crystalline lens of the eye.[22] He wrote also a treatise in thirty-seven chapters on gout. Many of the works of Rufus are lost, but fragments are preserved in other medical writings.

Marinus was an anatomist and physician who lived in the first and second centuries after Christ. Quintus was one of his pupils.

Marinus wrote twenty volumes on anatomy, of which Galen gives an abridgment and analysis. Galen says that Marinus was one of the restorers of anatomical science. Marinus investigated the glands and compared them to sponges, and he imagined that their function was to moisten and lubricate the surrounding structures. He discovered the glands of the intestines. He also wrote a commentary on the aphorisms of Hippocrates. It is uncertain if he is the Postumius Marinus who was physician to the younger Pliny.

Quintus was renowned in Rome in the first half of the second century after Christ. Like Galen he suffered from the jealousy and persecution of his professional rivals, who trumped up a charge against him of killing his patients, and he had to flee from the city. He was known as an expert anatomist, but published no medical writings. It has been stated by some of the writers on the history of medicine that Quintus was the tutor of Galen, but this statement is lacking in definite proof.

FOOTNOTES:

[21] For full description and plates see Dr. John Stewart Milne's "Surgical Instruments in Greek and Roman Times" (Clarendon Press, 1907).

[22] "Portal," vol. i, p. 74.

CHAPTER IX.

GALEN.

His life and works--His influence on Medicine.

Claudius Galenus, commonly known as Galen, has influenced the progress of medical science by his writings probably more than any other medical writer. His influence was paramount for fourteen centuries, and although he made some original contributions, his works are noteworthy mainly as an encyclopedia of the medical knowledge of his time and as a review of the work of his predecessors. There is a great deal of information in his books about his own life. He was born at Pergamos in A.D. 130 in the reign of Hadrian. His father was a scholar and his mother somewhat of a shrew. Galen, in his boyhood, learned much from his father's example and instruction, and at the age of 15 was taught by philosophers of the Stoic, Platonist, Peripatetic, and Epicurean schools. He became initiated, writes Dr. Moore, into "the idealism of Plato, the realism of Aristotle, the scepticism of the Epicureans, and the materialism of the Stoics." At the age of 17 he was destined for the profession of medicine by his father in consequence of a dream. He studied under the most eminent men of his day. He went to Smyrna to be a pupil of Pelops, the physician, and Albinus the platonist; to Corinth to study under Numesianus; to Alexandria for the lectures of Heraclianus; and to Cilicia, Phoenicia, Palestine, Crete, and Cyprus. At the age of 29 Galen returned from Alexandria to Pergamos (A.D. 158), and was appointed doctor to the School of Gladiators, and gained much distinction.

He went to Rome for the first time in A.D. 163-4, and remained for four years; and during this period he wrote on anatomy and on the teaching of Hippocrates and Plato. He acquired great fame as a practitioner and, if he had so desired, might have attended the Emperor; but it is probable that Galen thought that the office of physician to the Emperor might prevent him from leaving Rome if he wished to do so. He also gave public lectures and disputations, and was called not only the "wonder-speaker" but the "wonder-worker." His success gave rise to envy, and he was afraid of being poisoned by his less successful rivals. The reason why he left Rome is not certain, and the possible causes of his departure are discussed by Dr. Greenhill in the "Dictionary of Greek and Roman Biography and Mythology." A pestilence raged in Rome at this time, but it is unlikely that Galen would have deserted his patients for that reason. Probably he disliked Rome, and longed for his native place. He had been in Pergamos only a very short time when he was summoned to attend the Emperors Marcus Aurelius and L. Verus in Venetia. The latter died of apoplexy on his way home to Rome, and Galen followed Marcus Aurelius to the capital. The Emperor soon thereafter set out to prosecute the war on the Danube, and Galen was allowed to remain in Rome, as he had stated that such was the will. The Emperor's son Commodus was placed under the care of Galen during the father's absence, and at this time also (A.D. 170) Galen prepared the famous medicine theriaca for Marcus Aurelius, who took a small quantity daily. The Emperor Septimius Severus employed the same physician and the same medicine about thirty years afterwards. It is recorded that the philosopher Eudemius was successfully treated by Galen for a severe illness caused by an overdose of theriaca, and that the treatment employed was the same drug in small doses.

Galen stayed several years in Rome, and wrote and practised as on his former visit. He again returned to Pergamos, and probably was in Rome again at the end of the second century. It is certain he was still alive in the year 199, and probably lived in the reign of the Emperor Caracalla.

He was not only a great physician, but a man of wide culture in every way. In matters of religion he was a Monotheist. There was persecution of the Christians in his day, and it is likely that he came little into contact with the disciples of the new religion, and heard distorted accounts of it, but in one of his lost books, quoted by his Arabian biographers, Galen praises highly the love of virtue of the Christians.

He no doubt found the practice of medicine lucrative when he had gained pre-eminence, and it is recorded that he received ?50 for curing the wife of

Boetius, the Consul.

Galen wrote no less than five hundred treatises, large and small, mostly on medical subjects, but also on ethics, logic, and grammar. His style is good but rather diffuse, and he delights in quoting the ancient Greek philosophers. Before his time, as we have seen, there were disputes between the various medical sects. The disciples of Dogmatism and of Empiricism had been opposed to each other for several centuries, and the Eclectics, Pneumatists, and Episynthetics had arisen shortly before his time. Galen wrote against slavish attachment to any sect, but "in his general principles he may be considered as belonging to the Dogmatic sect, for his method was to reduce all his knowledge, as acquired by the observation of facts, to general theoretical principles. These principles he, indeed, professed to deduce from experience and observation, and we have abundant proofs of his diligence in collecting experience, and his accuracy in making observations; but still in a certain sense at least, he regards individual facts and the details of experience as of little value, unconnected with the principles which he had laid down as the basis of all medical reasoning. In this fundamental point, therefore, the method pursued by Galen appears to have been directly the reverse of that which we now consider as the correct method of scientific investigation; and yet, such is the force of natural genius, that in most instances he attained the ultimate object in view, although by an indirect path. He was an admirer of Hippocrates, and always speaks of him with the most profound respect, professing to act upon his principles, and to do little more than expound his doctrines, and support them by new facts and observations. Yet, in reality, we have few writers whose works, both as to substance and manner, are more different from each other than those of Hippocrates and Galen, the simplicity of the former being strongly contrasted with the abstruseness and refinement of the latter."[23]

A list of the various editions of Galen's works is given in Dr. Smith's "Dictionary of Greek and Roman Biography and Mythology" (1890 edition, vol. ii, pp. 210-12), and also the titles of the treatises classified according to the branch of medical science with which they deal, and it is convenient to follow this classification.

I.--WORKS ON ANATOMY AND PHYSIOLOGY.

Galen insisted upon the study of anatomy as essential, and in this respect was in conflict with the view held by the Methodists and the Empirics who believed that a physician could understand diseases without any knowledge of the exact structure of the body. His books on anatomy were originally fifteen in number. The last six of these are now extant only in an Arabic translation, two copies of which are preserved in the Bodleian Library at Oxford.

The directions he gives for dissection show that he was a master of the art. In dissecting out the portal vein and its ramifications, for instance, he advises that a probe should be inserted into the vein, and the point of the probe gradually advanced as the surrounding tissue is cut away, so that finally the minute branches are exposed; and he describes the use of the blowpipe, and other instruments used in dissection. He carried out the experiment of tying the iliac and axillary arteries in animals, and found that this procedure stopped the pulse in the leg and arm, but caused no serious symptoms, and he found that even the carotid arteries could be tied without causing death. He also pointed out that tying the carotid artery did not cause loss of voice, but that tying the artery carelessly so as to include the nerve had this effect. He was the first to describe the ductus arteriosus, and the three coats of the arteries.

It is highly improbable that Galen dissected human bodies in Rome, though he dissected a great variety of the lower animals. He writes that the doctors who attended Marcus Aurelius in the German wars dissected the dead bodies of the barbarians. The chief mistakes made by Galen as an anatomist were due to his assumption that what is true of the anatomy of a lower animal is true also when applied to man.

Galen greatly assisted the advance of physiology by recognizing that every part of the body exists for the purpose of performing a definite function. Aristotle, like Plato, had taught that "Nature makes nothing in vain," and Galen's philosophy was greatly influenced by the teaching of Aristotle. Galen regarded his work as "a religious hymn in honour of the Creator, who has given proof of His Omnipotence in creating everything perfectly conformable to its destination."

He regarded the structure of various parts, such as the hand and the membranes of the brain, as absolute perfection, although his idea of the human hand was derived from a study of the ape's, and he had no knowledge of the arachnoid membrane of the brain, but it would be unfair to criticize his conclusions because of his failure to recognize a few comparatively unimportant details. He discovered the function of the motor nerves by cutting them experimentally, and so producing paralysis of the muscles; the platysma, interossei, and popliteus muscles were first described by him. He was the greatest authority on the pulse, and he recognized that it consisted of a diastole (expansion) and a systole (contraction) with an interval after the diastole, and another after the systole. Aristotle thought that arteries contained air, but Galen taught that they contained blood, for, when an artery was wounded, blood gushed out. He was not far from the discovery of the circulation. He described the heart as having the appearance of a muscle, and considered it the source of natural heat, and the seat of violent passions. He knew well the anatomy of the human skeleton, and advised students to go to Alexandria where they might see and handle and properly study the bones. He recognized that inspiration is associated with enlargement of the chest, and imagined that air passed inside the skull through the cribriform plate of the ethmoid bone, and passed out by the same channel, carrying off humours from the brain into the nose. But some of this air remained and combined with the vital spirits in the anterior ventricles of the brain, and finally exuded from the fourth ventricle, the residence of the soul. Aristotle had taught that the heart was the seat of the soul, and the brain relatively unimportant.

II.--WORKS ON DIETETICS AND HYGIENE.

Galen was a strong advocate of exercises and gymnastics, and eulogizes hunting specially. He recommends cold baths for people in the prime of life. As old age is "cold and dry," this is to be treated with hot baths and the drinking of wine. He thought that wine was particularly suitable for the aged, and that old people required three meals a day, others two meals. He had a very high opinion of pork as an article of diet, and said that the strength of athletes could not be maintained without this form of food.

III.--ON PATHOLOGY.

Galen believed in the doctrine of the four elements, and his speculations led him into a belief in a further subdivision. "Fire is hot and dry; air is hot and moist; for the air is like a vapour; water is cold and moist, and earth is cold and dry." He held that there were three principles in man--spirits, solids, and humours--and eight temperaments ranging between health and disease and compatible with life. He retained a good deal of the teaching of the Pneumatic school, and believed that the pneuma was different from the soul, but the vehicle for the interaction of soul and body. From his theory of the action of the air through the nose on the contents of the ventricles of the brain is explained his use of sternutatories, and his belief in the efficacy of sneezing. Galen's classification of inflammations shows that his pathology was not nearly so accurate as his anatomy and physiology. He described (a) simple inflammation caused by excess of blood alone; (b) inflammation the result of excess of both pneuma and blood; (c) erysipelatous inflammation when yellow bile gains admission, and (d) scirrhous or cancerous when phlegm is present. He did good service by dividing the causes of disease into remote and proximate, the former subdivided into two classes--predisposing and exciting.

IV.--ON DIAGNOSIS.

He relied greatly on the doctrine of "critical days," which were thought to be influenced to some extent by the moon. His studies of the pulse were very useful to him in diagnosis. No doubt, he was an expert diagnostician mainly owing to his long, varied, and costly medical education, and his great natural powers of judgment. He asserted that with the help of the Deity he had never been wrong, but even his most ardent admirers would not be wanting in enthusiasm if they amended "never" into "hardly ever."

V.--ON PHARMACY, MATERIA MEDICA, AND THERAPEUTICS.

In these subjects Galen was not as proficient as Dioscorides, whose teaching he adopted with that of other medical authors. In Galen's works there are lengthy lists of compound medicines, several medicines being recommended for the same disease, and never with very marked confidence. He paid high prices for various nostrums, and, sad to relate, placed great faith in amulets, belief in which was general in his time, and nowhere held more strongly than in superstitious Rome. Medicines were classified by him according to their qualities, by which he meant, not their therapeutic effects, but their inherent dryness or moistness, coldness or heat. A medicine might be cold in the first degree, and not in the second degree. Paulus Aineta followed this strange and foolish doctrine of Galen very closely, as the following extracts from his book on Materia Medica will show:--

"Cistus (rock-rose).--It is an astringent shrub of gently cooling powers. Its leaves and shoots are so desiccative as to agglutinate wounds; but the flowers are of a more drying nature, being about the second degree; and hence, when drunk, they cure dysenteries and all kinds of fluxes."[24]

"Ferrum (iron).--When frequently extinguished in water, it imparts a considerable desiccative power to it. When drunk, therefore, it agrees with affections of the spleen."[25]

Many features, however, of Galen's teaching and practice of therapeutics are worthy of praise. He enunciated two fundamental principles: (1) That disease is something contrary to Nature, and is to be overcome by that which is contrary "to the disease itself"; and (2) that Nature is to be preserved by what has relation with Nature. He recognized that while the invading disease was to be repelled, the strength and constitution of the patient should be preserved, and that in all cases the cause of the disease was to be treated and not the symptoms. Strong remedies should not be used on weak patients.

VI.--SURGERY.

Galen conformed to the custom of the physicians in Rome, and did not practise surgery to any extent, although he used the lancet in phlebotomy, and defended this practice against the followers of Erasistratus in Rome. He is said to have resected a portion of the sternum for caries, and also to have ligatured the temporal artery.[26]

VII.--GYNECOLOGY.

Galen had little more than a superficial knowledge of this subject, and was quite ignorant of the surgery of diseases of women. He was not so well informed as Soranus was as to the anatomy of the uterus and its appendages, but deserves credit for having been better acquainted with the anatomy of the Fallopian tubes than his predecessors. He had erroneous views on the causation of displacements of the uterus. Several of the books inaccurately attributed to the authorship of Galen deal with the medical treatment of various minor ailments of women.

Galen was a man of wide culture, and one of his essays is written for the purpose of urging physicians to become acquainted with other branches of knowledge besides medicine. As a philosopher he has been quoted in company with Plato and Aristotle, and his philosophical writings were greatly used by Arabic authors. In philosophy, as in medicine, he had studied the teachings of the various schools of thought, and did not bind himself to any sect in particular. He disagreed with the Sceptics in their belief that no such thing as certainty was attainable, and it was his custom in cases of extreme difficulty to suspend his judgment; for instance, in reference to the nature of the soul, he wrote that he had not been able to come to a definite opinion.

Galen mentions the discreditable conduct of physicians at consultations. Sometimes several doctors would hold a consultation, and, apparently forgetting the patient for the time, would hold violent disputations. Their main object was to display their dialectical skill, and their arguments sometimes led to blows. These discreditable exhibitions were rather frequent in Rome in his time.

With Galen, as with Hippocrates, it is sometimes impossible to tell what works are genuine, and what are spurious. He seemed to think that he was the successor of Hippocrates, and wrote: "No one before me has given the true method of treating disease: Hippocrates, I confess, has heretofore shown the path, but as he was the first to enter it, he was not able to go as far as he wished.... He has not made all the necessary distinctions, and is often obscure, as is usually the case with ancients when they attempt to be concise. He says very little of complicated diseases; in a word, he has only sketched what another was to complete; he has opened the path, but has left it for a successor to enlarge and make it plain." Galen strictly followed Hippocrates in the latter's humoral theory of pathology, and also in therapeutics to a great extent.

It is a speculation of much interest how it was that Galen's views on Medicine received universal acceptance, and made him the dictator in this realm of knowledge for ages after his death. He was not precisely a genius, though a very remarkable man, and he established no sect of his own. The reason of his power lay in the fact that his writings supplied an encyclopaedic knowledge of the medical art down to his own time, with commentaries and additions of his own, written with great assurance and conveying an impression of finality, for he asserted that he had finished what Hippocrates had begun. The world was tired of political and philosophical strife, and waiting for authority. The wars of Rome had resulted in placing political power in the hands of one man, the Emperor; the disputations and bickerings of philosophers and physicians produced a similar result, and Galen, in the medical world was invested with the purple.

The effect, therefore, of Galen's writings was, at first, to add to and consolidate medical knowledge, but his influence soon became an obstacle to progress. Even in the sixteenth and seventeenth centuries, Galenism held almost undisputed sway.

The house of Galen stood opposite the Temple of Romulus in the Roman Forum. This temple, in A.D. 530, was consecrated by Pope Felix IV to the honour of the saints, Cosma and Damiano, two Arabian anargyri (unpaid physicians) who suffered martyrdom under Diocletian.

The date of Galen's death is not exactly known, but was probably A.D. 200.

FOOTNOTES:

[23] Dr. Bostock's "History of Medicine."

[24] "Paulus Aineta," vol. iii, p. 74.

[25] Ibid., p. 242.

[26] "Encyl. Brit.," Surgery.

CHAPTER X.

THE LATER ROMAN AND BYZANTINE PERIOD.

Beginning of Decline--Neoplatonism--Antyllus--Oribasius--Magnus-- Jacobus Psychristus--Adamantius--Meletius--Nemesius-- Alexander of Tralles--The Plague--Moschion--Paulus Aineta--Decline of Healing Art.

The death of Galen marks the beginning of the decline of medical science in ancient times, and this decline was contemporaneous with the overthrow of the Roman State. As everybody knows, the decline and fall of the Roman Empire resulted from the profligacy and incapacity of the emperors, luxurious living and vice among the people, tyranny of an overbearing soldiery at home, and the attacks of barbarian foes gradually increasing in strength. Rome fell quickly into the hands of the barbarians, and her power was broken. In A.D. 395, was founded the Byzantine Empire, also styled the East Roman, Greek, or Lower Empire, which lasted for more than a thousand years, and took its name from the capital, Byzantium or Constantinople. In this empire medical science maintained a feeble and sickly existence. During this Byzantine Period there were a few physicians of note, but they were mainly commentators, and medical science retrograded rather than progressed.

Neoplatonism exerted a powerful influence upon the healing art. It was founded by Plotinus, and was for three centuries a formidable rival to Christianity. The Neoplatonists believed that man could intuitively know the absolute by a faculty called Ecstasy. Neoplatonism is a term which covers a very wide range of varying thought; essentially, it was a combination of philosophy and religion, arising from the intellectual movement in Alexandria. It covered a great deal of mysticism, magic and spiritualism, and the followers of the system, as it developed, became believers in the efficacy of certain exercises and symbols to cure diseases. They entered as Kingsley wrote, "the fairy land of ecstasy, clairvoyance, insensibility to pain, cures produced by the effect of what we now call mesmerism. They are all there, these modern puzzles, in those old books of the long bygone seekers for wisdom." It is wonderful how mankind in their pursuit of knowledge seem to have progressed in a circle.

The influence which Christianity exerted upon the investigation of medical science during the early centuries of our era will be considered at length in a subsequent chapter.

Antyllus was perhaps the greatest surgeon of antiquity. He lived before the end of the fourth century A.D., for he is quoted by Oribasius, but is not mentioned by Galen. The time in which he lived was about the year A.D. 300. He was a voluminous writer, but his works have perished except for quotations by later writers. The fragments of his writings were collected and published in 1799. Antyllus performed an operation for aneurism, which consisted in laying open the sac, turning out the clots, securing the vessels above and below, and allowing the wound to heal by granulation. As this operation was performed without anesthetics or antiseptics it was attended with great mortality, and the risk of secondary hemorrhage was very great. Antyllus had operations for the cure of stammering, for cataract, and for the treatment of contractures by the method of tenotomy. He also removed enlarged glands of the neck. It was part of the practice of Antyllus to ligature arteries before cutting them, a method which was subsequently "rediscovered" owing to neglect of the study of the history of medicine. He gave directions for avoiding the carotid artery and internal jugular vein in operations upon the neck.

A fragment of the writings of Antyllus is preserved by Paulus Aineta,[27] and shows the quality of the work done in bygone ages. It is his description of the operation of tracheotomy, and runs as follows:--

"When we proceed to perform this operation we must cut through some part of the windpipe, below the larynx, about the third or fourth ring; for to divide the whole would be dangerous. This place is commodious, because it is not covered with any flesh, and because it has no vessels situated near the divided part. Therefore, bending the head of the patient backward, so that the windpipe may come more forward to the view, we make a transverse section between two of the rings, so that in this case not the cartilage but the membrane which unites the cartilages together, is divided. If the operator be a little timid, he may first stretch the skin with a hook and divide it; then, proceeding to the windpipe, and separating the vessels, if any are in the way, he may make the incision." This operation had been proposed by Asclepiades about three hundred years before the time of Antyllus.

Oribasius was born at Pergamos, the birthplace of Galen, about A.D. 326. He studied under Zenon, who lectured and practised at Alexandria, and was expelled by the bishop, but afterwards reinstated by command of the Emperor Julian (A.D. 361). When Julian was kept in confinement in Asia Minor,

Oribasius became acquainted with him, and they were soon close friends. When Julian was raised to the rank of Caesar, Oribasius accompanied him into Gaul. During this journey Oribasius, at the request of his patron, made an epitome of the writings of Galen, and then extended the work by including a collection of the writings of all preceding medical authors. When this work was finally completed it consisted of seventy books under the title "Collecta Medicinalia." He wrote also for his friend and biographer Eunapius two books on diseases and their treatment, and treatises on anatomy and on the works of Galen. He earned for himself the title of the Ape of Galen. In the "Life of Oribasius," by Eunapius, we find that Julian created Oribasius Qutor of Constantinople, but after the death of Julian, Oribasius was exiled, and practised among the "barbarians," attaining great fame. In his exile he married a rich woman of good family, and to one of his sons, Eustathius by name, he addressed an abridgment of his first great book, the smaller work being called the "Synopsis." He ultimately returned from exile, and again reached a very honourable position, to which he was well entitled in virtue of the great fortitude with which he had borne adversity.

An edition of Oribasius was published at Paris between 1851 and 1876, in six volumes, by Daremberg and Bussemaker, under the patronage of the French Government. The authors of this edition took infinite pains to show the sources from which the writings of Oribasius had been derived, chief of which were the original writings of Galen, Hippocrates, Soranus, Rufus, and Antyllus. Oribasius was almost entirely a compiler, but also did some original work. To him is due the credit of describing the drum of the ear and the salivary glands. He described also the strange disease called lycanthropy, a form of insanity in which the patient thinks himself a wolf, and leaves his home at night to wander amongst the tombs.

Oribasius was held to be the wisest man of his time. There was something very charming in his manner and conversation, and the barbarians considered him as little less than a god.

Magnus, a native of Mesopotamia, was a pupil of Zenon and lectured at

Alexandria. He was famous for his eloquence and dialectical skill, and wrote a book on "Urine" which is referred to by Theophilus.

Jacobus Psychristus was a famous physician who practised at Constantinople, A.D. 457-474. He was called "the Saviour" because of the great success of his treatment.

Adamantius of Alexandria both taught and practised medicine. He was a Jewish physician who was expelled from Alexandria in A.D. 415, and settled in Constantinople.

Meletius was a Christian monk who lived in the fourth century, according to some authorities, but it is probable that he belonged to a later period, the sixth or seventh century. He wrote on the nature of man, but the book is of no value as a contribution to physiology.

Nemesius, Bishop of Emissa, at the end of the fourth century wrote a book called "De Natura Hominis," and came very close to two important discoveries, namely, the functions of the bile and the circulation of the blood. Of the former, he wrote, "The yellow bile is constituted both for itself and for other purposes; for it contributes to digestion and promotes the expulsion of the excrements; and therefore it is in a manner one of the nutritive organs, besides imparting a sort of heat to the body, like the vital power. For these reasons, therefore, it seems to be made for itself; but, inasmuch as it purges the blood, it seems to be made in a manner for this also."[28]

With reference to the circulation of the blood, Nemesius wrote: "The motion of the pulse (called also the vital power) takes its rise from the heart and chiefly from its left ventricle. The artery is with great vehemence dilated and contracted, by a sort of constant harmony and order, the motion commencing at the heart. While it is dilated it draws with force the thinner part of the blood from the neighbouring veins, the exhalation or vapour of which blood becomes the aliment for the vital spirit. But while it is contracted it exhales whatever fumes it has through the whole body and by secret passages, as the heart throws out whatever is fuliginous through the mouth and nose by expiration."[29]

This book was first translated into English in 1636.

Nemesius also wrote on religion and philosophy. In regard to his medical writings, although he did not go far enough to anticipate the discovery of Harvey, his contribution to medical science was remarkable.

茴 ius was born in Mesopotamia and lived at the end of the fifth or the beginning of the sixth century. He studied at Alexandria, and settled at Constantinople, where he attained to the honour of court chamberlain, and physician to the Emperor Justinian. He was the first notable physician to profess Christianity. In compounding medicines, he recommended that the following prayer should be repeated in a low voice: "May the God of Abraham, the God of Isaac, and the God of Jacob deign to bestow upon this medicament such and such virtues." To extract a piece of bone sticking in the throat, the physician should call out loudly: "As Jesus Christ drew Lazarus from the grave, and as Jonah came out of the whale, thus Blasius, the martyr and servant of God, commands, 'Bone, come up or go down.'"

茴 ius wrote the "Sixteen Books on Medicine," and these contain original matter, but are of value mainly as being a compilation of the medical knowledge of his time. He was the first writer to mention certain Eastern drugs, such as cloves and camphor, and had a great knowledge of the spells and charms used in the East, more especially by the Egyptian Christians. All the nostrums, amulets and charms that were used at the time are enumerated, and display a gloomy picture of the superstition and ignorance that prevailed. The surgical and gyn 鎐 ological sections of the writings of 茴 ius are, in most parts, excellent. He treated cut arteries by twisting or tying, and advised the irrigation of wounds with cold water. In the operation of lithotomy he recommended that the blade of the knife should be guarded by a tube. He used the seton and the cautery, which was much in vogue in his day, especially in cases of paralysis. He quotes Archigenes, who wrote: "I should not at all hesitate to make an eschar in the nape of the neck, where the spinal marrow takes its rise, two on each side of it ... and if the ulcers continue running a good while, I should not doubt of a perfect recovery."

Alexander of Tralles lived from A.D. 525 to 605. He was the son of a physician, and one of five brothers, who were all distinguished for scholarship. He studied philosophy as well as medicine, and travelled in France, Spain, and Italy to extend his knowledge. He took up permanent residence in Rome, and became very celebrated. When he became too old to continue active practice, he found leisure to write twelve books on medical diseases, following to some extent the teaching of Galen. The style of these books is elegant, and his description of diseases accurate. Alexander of Tralles was the first to open the jugular vein in disease, and employed iron and other useful remedies, but he lived in superstitious times, and was very credulous. For epilepsy, he recommended a piece of sail from a wrecked vessel, worn round the arm for seven weeks.[30] For colic, he recommended the heart of a lark attached to the right thigh, and for pain in the kidneys an amulet depicting Hercules overcoming a lion. To exorcise gout, he used incantations, these being either oral or written on a thin sheet of gold during the waning of the moon. Writing a suitable inscription on an olive leaf, gathered before sunrise, was his specific for ague. Alexander appears at times to have doubted the efficacy of such remedies as amulets, for he explains that his rich patients would not submit to rational treatment, and it was necessary, therefore, to use other methods reputed to be curative.

In the age of Justinian great scourges devastated the world. In A.D. 526 Antioch was destroyed by an earthquake, and it is said that 250,000 people perished, but the most dreadful visitation on mankind was the great plague which raged in A.D. 542 and the following years, and, as Gibbon writes, "depopulated the earth in the time of Justinian and his successors." Procopius, who was versed in medicine, was the historian of the period. This fell disease began between the Serbonian bog and the eastern channel of the Nile. "From thence, tracing as it were a double path, it spread to the east, over Syria, Persia, and the Indies, and penetrated to the west, along the coast of Africa, and over the continent of Europe. In the spring of the second year, Constantinople, during three or four months, was visited by the pestilence; and Procopius, who observed its progress and symptoms with the eyes of a physician, has emulated the skill and diligence of Thucydides in the latter's description of the plague of Athens. The infection was sometimes announced by the visions of a distempered fancy, and the victim despaired as soon as he had heard the menace and felt the stroke of an invisible spectre. But the greater number, in their beds, in the streets, in their usual occupation, were surprised by a slight fever, so slight, indeed, that neither the pulse nor the colour of the patient gave any signs of the approaching danger. The same, the next, or the succeeding day, it was declared by the swelling of the glands, particularly those of the groin, of the armpits, and under the ear; and when these buboes or tumours were opened they were found to contain a coal, or black substance, of the size of a lentil. If they came to a first swelling and suppuration, the patient was saved by this kind and natural discharge of the morbid humour. But if they continued hard and dry, a mortification quickly ensued, and the fifth day was commonly the term of his life. The fever was often accompanied with lethargy or delirium; the bodies of the sick were covered with black pustules or carbuncles, the symptoms of immediate death; and in the constitutions too feeble to produce an eruption, the vomiting of blood was followed by a mortification of the bowels. To pregnant women the plague was generally mortal; yet one infant was drawn alive from its dead mother, and three mothers survived the loss of their infected foetus. Youth was the most perilous season: and the female sex was less susceptible than the male; but every rank and profession was attacked with indiscriminate rage, and many of those who escaped were deprived of their speech, without being secure from a return of the disorder. The physicians of Constantinople were zealous and skilful, but their art was baffled by the various symptoms and pertinacious vehemence of the disease; the same remedies were productive of contrary effects and the event capriciously disappointed their prognostics of death or recovery. The order of funerals and the right of sepulchres were confounded; those who were left without friends or servants lay unburied in the streets, or in their desolate houses; and a magistrate was authorized to collect the promiscuous heaps of dead bodies, to transport them by land or water, and to inter them in deep pits beyond the precincts of the city.... No facts have been preserved to sustain an account, or even a conjecture, of the number that perished in this extraordinary mortality. I only find, that during three months 5,000, and at length 10,000, persons died each day at Constantinople; that many cities of the East were left vacant, and that in several districts of Italy the harvest and the vintage withered on the ground."[31]

The spread of disease from East to West was again exemplified in the Middle Ages, in the time of the Crusades, when the Crusaders carried home diseases to their native lands. The Knights of St. John, it is interesting to observe, superintended hospitals at home, and wore the white dress which in earlier times had distinguished the Asclepiades.

Moschion probably lived in the sixth century, and was a specialist in diseases of women. His writings were studied when Soranus was forgotten, but in course of time it was discovered that Moschion's work was nothing but an abbreviated translation of the works of Soranus. "Further, it is held by Weber and Ermerins that even the original Moschion is not based directly on Soranus, but on a work on diseases of women written in the fourth century by Casius Aurelianus, who in his turn drew from Soranus.... It is interesting to follow the history of this book through its various stages in the light of these different editions, and we would suggest that the first Latin version, for the use of Latin-speaking matrons and midwives, was produced before the fall of the Western Empire in the fifth century; its Greek sister just fits in with the development of Eastern or Greek-speaking Empire at Constantinople in the sixth century; and the version in barbarous Latin points to a later period, when learning was beginning to make way again in Western Europe."[32] Moschion's book is a catechism consisting of 152 questions and answers.

Paulus Aineta was the last, and one of the most famous, of the Greek physicians. He was born probably in the seventh century in the island ofAina, but there is some doubt as to the exact period in which he lived. He quotes Alexander of Tralles, and therefore lived at a later period than they did, either in the sixth or seventh century. The works of Paulus are compilations, but reveal the skill and learning of the author. He wrote several books, but only one, and that the principal, remains, and is known by the title of "De Re Medica Libri Septem." Dr. Adams, of Banchory, translated this book for the Sydenham Society, and the introduction shows the scope of the work: "In the first book you will find everything that relates to hygiene, and to the preservation from, and correction of, distempers peculiar to the various ages, reasons, temperaments, and so forth; also the powers and use of the different articles of food, as is set forth in the chapter of contents. In the second is explained the whole doctrine of fevers, an account of certain matters relating to them being premised, such as excrementitious discharges, critical days, and other appearances, and concluding with certain symptoms which are the concomitants of fevers. The third book relates to topical affections, beginning from the crown of the head and descending down to the nails of the feet, and so on. Briefly, the fourth book treats of external diseases; the fifth, of wounds and bites from venomous animals; the sixth book is the most important and is devoted to surgery, and contains original observations, and the seventh book contains an account of the properties of medicines." Paulus wrote a famous book on obstetrics, which is now lost, but it gained for him among the Arabs the title of "the accoucheur."

The sixth book on surgery, as has justly been observed by Adams, "contains the most complete system of operative surgery which has come down to us from ancient times." Many important surgical principles are enunciated, such, for instance, as local depletion as against general, and the merit of a free external incision. He first described varicose aneurism, and performed the operation of bronchotomy as described by Antyllus. He favoured the lateral operation for removal of stone from the bladder, and amputated the cancerous breast by crucial incision. He also had an operation, like that of Antyllus, for the cure of aneurism. In brief, Paulus performed many of the operations that are practised at the present day. He travelled in the practice of his calling, and not only had great fame in the Byzantine Empire and in Arabia in his lifetime, but exercised great influence for some centuries. His writings inspired Albucassis, one of the few surgeons and teachers of the

Middle Ages.

After the time of Paulus ineta the practice of medicine and surgery suffered a very rapid decline, and for five centuries no progress was made. The Middle Ages form a dark and melancholy period in the history of medicine, and we have to come to comparatively recent times before we find the skill and knowledge of the Ancients equalled, while it is only at the present day that they are rapidly being excelled.

FOOTNOTES:

[27] "De re Med.," vi, 33.

[28] C. 28, p. 260, ed. Matth.

[29] C. 24, p. 242.

[30] Lib. 1, c. 20.

[31] Gibbon, "The Decline and Fall of the Roman Empire."

[32] Barbour, Edinburgh Medical Journal, vol. xxxiv, p. 331.

CHAPTER XI.

INFLUENCE OF CHRISTIANITY ON ALTRUISM AND THE HEALING ART.

Essenes--Cabalists and Gnostics--Object of Christ's Mission--Stoics--Constantine and Justinian--Gladiatorial Games--Orphanages--Support of the Poor--Hospitals--Their Foundation--Christianity and Hospitals--Fabiola--Christian Philanthropy--Demon Theories of Disease receive the Church's Sanction--Monastic Medicine--Miracles of Healing--St. Paul--St. Luke--Proclus--Practice of Anatomy denounced--Christianity the prime factor in promoting Altruism.

The sect of the Essenes embraced part of the teaching of Christianity among their other beliefs. They conceived that the Almighty had to be propitiated by signs and symbols. Words, they considered, were the direct gift of God to man, and, therefore, signs representing words were of great avail. Hence arose the use of amulets and cabalistic signs, or, rather, the common use, for they had been in evidence long prior to the foundation of this sect. Amulets were worn on the person. The Jews had phylacteries or bits of parchment on which were written passages from the Scriptures. In the first century after Christ, Jews, Pythagoreans, Essenes, and various sects of mystics combined and formed the Cabalists and Gnostics. Their creed embraced the magic of the Persians, the dreams of the Asclepiads, the numbers of Pythagoras, and the theory of atoms of Democritus. The Sophists of Alexandria actually regarded magic as a science. A section of the early Christians were Gnostics, and were imbued with the philosophy of the Orientals. According to the beliefs of the Cabalists and Gnostics, demons were the cause of disease. These sects interrogated evil spirits to find out where they lurked, and exorcised them with the help of charms and talismans. Various geometric figures and devices were held to have power against evil spirits. One of these figures was the device of two triangles interlaced thus [Symbol: David's Star]. This was used as a symbol of God, not only by Cabalists and Gnostics, but also by Jews. The great majority of the early Christians opposed the Gnostics, and repudiated and abhorred their strange mixture of the Christian religion with Eastern philosophy.

Christ came into the world at a time when the evils of slavery were probably at their worst. He did not directly condemn slavery, and the reason of this is to be found in the study of the nature of His mission. He came to regenerate the individual, and not, primarily, society. "His language in innumerable similes showed that He believed that those principles He taught would only be successful after long periods of time and gradual development. Most of His figures and analogies in regard to 'the Kingdom of God' rest upon the idea of slow and progressive growth or change. He undoubtedly saw that the only true renovation of the world would come, not through reforms of institutions or governments, but through individual change of character, effected by the same power to which Plato appealed--the love-power--but a love exercised towards Himself as a perfect and Divine model. It was the 'Kingdom of God' in the soul which should bring on the kingdom of God in human society.... And yet ultimately this Christian system will be found at the basis of all these great movements of progress in human history. But it began by aiming at the individual, and not at society; and aiming alone at an entire change of the affectional and moral tendencies."[33]

The moral teaching of the Stoics, second only to that of the Christian religion, had an effect in preparing the way for the introduction of humane principles of treatment for the bond and the oppressed. But the Stoics, like many of the Christians, did not always make their actions accord with their principles. Seneca tells of a Stoic who amused himself by feeding his fish with pieces of his mutilated slaves. Juvenal, who wrote when Stoicism was at the height of its influence, asks "how a slave could be a man," and Gaius, the Stoical jurist, in the reign of Marcus Aurelius, classes slaves with animals.

Constantine, in his own character, did not display the beauties of the Christian religion, though his advisers who framed his laws acted under the influence of Christian teaching. This emperor passed laws in reference to slavery. He wrote to an archbishop: "It has pleased me for a long time to establish that, in the Christian Church, masters can give liberty to their slaves, provided they do it in presence of all the assembled people with the assistance of Christian priests, and provided that, in order to preserve the memory of the fact, some written document informs where they sign as parties or as witnesses." In pagan times there was a somewhat similar system of a master being able to redeem a slave and register the redemption in one of the temples.

The laws of Justinian, influenced largely by the teaching of Christianity, did a great deal to relieve the burdens of slavery. "We do not transfer persons from a free condition into a servile--we have so much at heart to raise slaves to liberty." In the words of one of the Early Fathers of the Church, "No

Christian is a slave; those born again are all brothers."

Gladiatorial Games were condemned by the Stoics, but these philosophers did not influence the common people. Constantine, in the year before his acceptance of Christianity, gave a multitude of prisoners as prey to the wild beasts of the arena. In A.D. 325 he promulgated this law: "Bloody spectacles, in our present state of tranquillity and domestic peace, do not please us; wherefore we order that all gladiators be prohibited from carrying on their profession." Human sacrifices, which at one time took place in Rome, even in the time of Pliny and Seneca, were abolished under the same influence as checked gladiatorial sports.

Constantine passed laws against the licentious plays and spectacles which flourished in Greece and Rome in pagan times.

Seneca wrote: "Monstrous offspring we destroy; children too, if weak and unnaturally formed from birth, we drown. It is not anger, but reason, thus to separate the useless from the sound."[34] Julius Paulus, a Stoic, in the time of the Emperor Severus (A.D. 222), held that the mother who procured abortion, starved her child, or exposed it to die, was, in each case, equally guilty of murder. The Christian Fathers, in opposing these evils, were acting in accordance with the teaching of their founder, and they incessantly condemned these evil practices, and with greater and more far-reaching power than the Stoics. Although the Stoics anticipated many of the reforms of the Christians, Stoicism never had any penetrating effect on the masses of the people, and differed in this respect from Christianity. The chief obstacle to the prevention of the exposure of children was the great amount of pauperism which prevailed in the Roman Empire, and Christian emperors and councils had no choice but to allow many of these unfortunate children to be taken as slaves, rather than that they should perish from cold and hunger, or be torn by ravenous beasts. The pagan emperors, it is true, had done something to found orphanages, but these institutions were not common until the Middle Ages. Trajan in A.D. 100 supported 5,000 children at the expense of the State, and endowments were created by him for this purpose.

Hadrian, Antoninus, and Marcus Aurelius made similar benefactions, and Pliny endowed a charity for poor children.

In the pre-Christian period, social clubs existed for the purpose of people having meals together, helping one another, and providing burial funds. The Emperor Julian condemned the Christians for supporting not only their own poor, but also poor strangers outside their faith. For ages the Church took charge of the poor. Her enemies said that as much pauperism was created as was relieved, and, no doubt, as is usual in the distribution of charity, the good done was not unmixed with evil.

HOSPITALS.

With reference to the important question of the foundation of hospitals, there are two opposing opinions--one, attributing their foundation almost entirely to Christianity,[35] and the other denying to Christianity any pre-eminent influence.[36] The truth lies between these two conflicting views, but nearer to the statement of Mr. Brace than of Mr. McCabe. The truths and influences of Christianity, in the mind of the latter author, are obscured by the many errors of the Church, especially in the Early and Middle Ages; and it is of the utmost importance to distinguish, where necessary, between the teaching of the Founder of Christianity as disclosed in the New Testament, and the teaching of the Church which made many very evident errors, and whose practice soon became different from that inculcated by its Founder, so that at times the Christianity of the Church was as different from Christ's teaching as the vine of Sodom from the grapes of Eshcol. The fact that Christianity emerged from this eclipse points to it as something more than a humanly devised system.

In very early times, the sick were allowed to remain at the temples for the treatment of their diseases, and medical students also attended for instruction. This system was the hospital system of later times, although the temples were not hospitals in the present sense of the word. The system in vogue in the temples of Aculapius in Greece and Rome has already been described in this book, but the temples of Saturn served the same purpose in Egypt four thousand years before Christ. Professor Ebers of Leipzig, a high authority on the subject, says that Heliopolis undoubtedly had a clinique in connection with the temple. The Emperor Asoka founded many hospitals in Hindustan, and Buddhists and Mohammedans both possessed hospitals ("Encyclopedia Britannica").

Patients were attracted to temples, not only by receiving the services of the priest-physicians, but also in the superstitious belief that special virtue attached to the precincts of sacred buildings. Thus, in the temples of Aculapius, sick people tried to get as near to the altar as possible. "It may fairly be surmised that the disuse of these temples in Christian times made the necessity of hospitals more apparent, and so led to their institution, in much the same way as in this country the suppression of monasteries, which had largely relieved the indigent poor, made the necessity of poor laws immediately evident."[37] During Hadrian's reign the first notice of a military hospital appears.

The iatria, or tabern?medic? described by Galen and others, were not for in-patients, but of the nature of dispensaries for the reception of out-patients. Seneca refers to valetudinaria, rooms set aside for the sick in large private houses. The first hospital in Rome in Christian times was founded by Fabiola, a wealthy lady, at the end of the fourth century. Attached to it was a convalescent home in the country. Pulcheria, later, built and endowed several hospitals at Constantinople, and these subsequently increased in number. Pauline abandoned wealth and social position and went to Jerusalem, and there established a hospital and sisterhood under the direction of St. Jerome. St. Augustine founded a hospital at Hippo. McCabe states justly: "In the new religious order a philanthropic heroism was evolved that was certainly new to Europe. In the whole story of Stoicism there is no figure like that of a Catherine of Sienna sucking the sores of a leper, or a Vincent de Paul." It appears evident that Christianity was an important factor in the foundation of hospitals and charitable institutions, not directly, but from its beneficent influence on the character of individuals; and the Roman Church, in this respect, acted in conformity with the teachings of the Christian faith.

Of greater importance is the consideration of the influence of Christianity, and of the Church, on the investigation and elimination of disease. In this matter the Church deserves the severest censure. It is no exaggeration to say that she hindered the scientific progress of the world for centuries. She applied to the explanation of the causation of disease, the demon theories inherited from Egypt, Persia, and the East. The Bible itself reflects the views on demonology current at the time of the events recorded. If demons were the cause of disease, logically the treatment of diseases should have been in the hands of priests, not of physicians. The priests held that they were the proper people to interpret the will of the Almighty; diseases were direct dispensations of Providence.

"It is demons," says Origen, "which produce famine, unfruitfulness, corruptions of the air, and pestilence. They hover concealed in clouds, in the lower atmosphere, and are attracted by the blood and incense which the heathen offer to them as gods."[38] "All diseases of Christians," wrote Augustine, "are to be ascribed to these demons: chiefly do they torment fresh-baptized Christians, yea! even the guiltless new-born infants." Hippocrates, long before the Christian era, wrote with great wisdom in reference to the so-called sacred diseases: "To me it appears that such affections are just as much divine as all others are, and that no one disease is either more divine or more human than another; but all are alike divine, for each has its own nature, and no one arises without a natural cause."[39]

The devil might be driven out in disgust, it was thought, by the use of disgusting materials--ordure, the grease made from executed criminals, the livers of toads, the blood of rats, and so on. The same belief in demoniacal possession led to the most inhuman treatment of lunatics, and the Church in this respect is put to shame when we compare its action with the wiser and more humane practice of the Moors. This belief helped to strangle medical progress for centuries, and is directly attributable to the Church. As late as 1583, the Jesuit fathers at Vienna boasted that they had cast out 12,642 devils. That God dispenses both health and disease is a very different belief from that involved in "demoniacal possession." Travellers in remote parts of the East at the present day tell of alleged cases of demoniacal possession, but investigation does not reveal any difference between these cases and epilepsy or acute mania.

In the first centuries of the Christian era men demanded overt signs of the favour of God, and the objects of veneration kept in the churches and monasteries were held to be capable of curing disease. The Latin Church had either a saint or a relic of a saint to cure nearly every ill that flesh is heir to. St. Apollonia was invoked against toothache; St. Avertin against lunacy; St. Benedict against stone; St. Clara against sore eyes; St. Herbert in hydrophobia; St. John in epilepsy; St. Maur in gout; St. Pernel in ague; St. Genevieve in fever; St. Sebastian in plague; St. Ottila for diseases of the head; St. Blazius for the neck; St. Laurence and St. Erasmus for the body; St. Rochus and St. John for diseases of the legs and feet. St. Margaret was invoked for diseases of children and the dangers of childbirth.

What the influence of Christ's life on earth on the medical art of His time was is a difficult question. It must be remembered that He came to save the souls and not the bodies of men, not to rapidly alter social conditions nor to teach science. The eternal life of man was the subject of transcendent importance, and it is no doubt true that many of the early Christians neglected their bodies for the cure of their souls. As against this, the gospel of love taught that all men are brothers, both bond and free, and this led to mutual help in physical suffering, and to the foundation of charitable institutions. In the times of persecution of the Christians many of them welcomed suffering and death as the portal to eternal bliss.

It has been asserted that the miraculous cures wrought by Christ for His own purposes were an intimation to His followers to neglect the ordinary means of natural cure, and that this placed a Christian doctor in the position of having to abandon his calling. This is not so. To St. Luke--a Christian physician and the writer of the third Gospel and the Acts of the Apostles--the performance by Christ of miracles of healing presented no difficulties, for he was the travelling medical adviser of St. Paul, and accompanied him on three journeys, from Troas to Philippi, from Philippi to Jerusalem, and from Caesarea to Rome (A.D. 62). St. Paul wrote: "For we would not, brethren, have you ignorant of our trouble which came to us in Asia, that we were pressed out of measure, above strength, insomuch that we despaired even of life, but we had the sentence of death in ourselves, that we should not trust in ourselves, but in God, which raiseth the dead: who delivered us from so great a death, and doth deliver: in whom we trust that He will yet deliver us." St. Paul exercised faith, but also used the means of cure prescribed by "the beloved physician." In a very scholarly book published by the Dublin University Press in 1882, the Rev. W. K. Hobart, LL.D., shows that St. Luke was acquainted with the technical medical terms of the Greek medical writers. St. Luke was an Asiatic Greek. Dr. Hobart writes: "Finally, it should not be left out of account that, in any illness from which he might be suffering, there was no one to whom St. Paul would be likely to apply with such confidence as to St. Luke, for it is probable that, in the whole extent of the Roman Empire, the only Christian physician at this time was St. Luke." In later years the pretence of performing miracles to cure diseases had a great effect in advancing superstition and retarding scientific investigation.

Tacitus and Suetonius record miracles alleged to have been performed by Vespasian. He is said to have anointed the eyes of a blind man at Alexandria with the royal spittle, and to have restored his sight. Another case was that of a man who had lost the use of his hands, and Vespasian touched them with his foot and thus restored their function. It is interesting to follow the career of Proclus, the last rector of the Neoplatonic School, "whose life," says Gibbon, "with that of his scholar Isidore, composed by two of their most learned disciples, exhibits a most deplorable picture of the second childhood of human reason." By long fasting and prayer Proclus pretended to possess the supernatural power of expelling all diseases.

The priests of the Church denounced the practice of Anatomy, and so changed the progress made by the Alexandrian School, and by men like Galen, into the ignorance of a thousand years. The body was the temple of the Holy Ghost, and should not therefore be desecrated by dissection. "Strangers' rests" and hospitals were connected with the monasteries, and were exceedingly useful, notably in the time of the Crusades, but these Church institutions were in a very insanitary condition, for the maxim that cleanliness is next to godliness had little application among the religious orders of the Middle Ages. Dr. Walsh attempts to show that the Reformers blackened the fair fame of the Church they had left, and states that it is to "this unfortunate state of affairs, and not real opposition on the part of the Popes to science," that we owe the belief in "the supposed opposition between the Church and Science."[40] That the Popes did something to foster medical science in a spasmodic kind of way, that papal physicians were appointed and that the Church exercised control over some seats of learning may be freely admitted. That the monasteries preserved some of the Latin classics that they were not all corrupt, and that all monks were not ignorant and idle, are facts beyond dispute. No doubt, too, the enemies of Christianity have overstated their case, but when all is said, the fact remains that the Church enjoyed great opportunities for promoting knowledge and investigating disease, and failed to avail itself of them to such an extent that for ages no real progress was made. This is certainly not an extreme opinion. It would be nearer the truth to say that not only was no progress made, but that the advances made by Hippocrates, by the school of Alexandria, by Celsus, and by Galen, were lost.

In conclusion, in spite of the dreadful blunders and perversions of the Church in the Early and Middle Ages, and the partial eclipse which Christianity suffered, the teaching of its Founder slowly but surely ended the harsh and cruel ways of the pagans, and was the prime factor in promoting the altruism of later times, of which medical knowledge and medical service form a very important part.

FOOTNOTES:

[33] "Gesta Christi; or a History of Human Progress under Christianity," by C. Loring Brace, fourth edition, pp. 33, 34.

[34] "De Ira," i, 15.

[35] Vide "Gesta Christi," Brace.

[36] Vide "The Bible in Europe," Joseph McCabe.

[37] "Smith's Dictionary of Greek and Roman Antiquity."

[38] Origen, "Contra Celsum," lib. vii.

[39] Adams's translation "Hippoc.," vol. i, p. 216.

[40] "The Popes and Science: The History of the Papal Relations to Science during the Middle Ages, and down to our own Time," J. J. Walsh, M.D., 1911.

CHAPTER XII.

GYMNASIA AND BATHS.

Gymnastics--Vitruvius--Opinions of Ancient Physicians on Gymnastics--The Athletes--The Baths--Description of Baths at Pompeii--Therm?-Baths of Caracalla.

GYMNASTICS.

Gymnastics were held in such high repute in ancient Greece that physical training occupied as much time in the education of boys as all their other studies, and was continued through life with modifications to suit the altering requirements of age and occupation. The Greeks fully recognized that mental culture could not reach its highest perfection if the development of the body were neglected. Lucian attributes not only the bodily grace of the Ancient Greeks, but also their mental pre-eminence, to the gymnastic exercises which they practised. They were also an important factor in the excellence of Greek sculpture, and probably the most important part of their medical treatment.

Unfortunately the baths of the Romans and the gymnasia of the Greeks became in time the haunts of the lazy and voluptuous. The gymnastic exercises of the Greeks date from very early times, and at first were of a warlike nature, and not reduced to a system. Each town possessed a gymnasium, and three very important ones were situated at Athens.

Vitruvius describes the general plan of an ancient gymnasium. It comprised a great stadium capable of accommodating a vast concourse of spectators, many porticoes where athletes exercised and philosophers and sages held discussions and lectured, walks and shady groves, and baths and anointing rooms. The buildings, in true Grecian fashion, were made very beautiful, being adorned with statues and works of art, and situated in pleasant surroundings.

Up to the age of 16 boys were instructed in gymnastics, in music and in grammar, and from 16 to 18 in gymnastics alone. The laws of Solon regulated the use of the gymnasia, and for very many years these laws were strictly enforced. It appears that married women did not attend the gymnasia, and unmarried women only in some parts of Greece, such as Sparta, but this custom was relaxed in later years.

The office of Gymnasiarch (Superintendent of Gymnasia) was one of great honour, but involved also a great deal of expense to the holder of the office. He wore a purple cloak and white shoes. Officers were appointed to supervise the morals and conduct of the boys and youths, and the Gymnasiarch had power to expel people whose teaching or example might be injurious to the young.

Galen relates that the chief teachers of the gymnasia were capable of prescribing suitable exercises, and thus had powers of medical supervision.

Before exercises were commenced, the body was anointed, and fine sand or dust applied. Regulation of the diet was considered of very great importance.

The games of the gymnasia were many and various, including games of ball, tug-of-war, top-spinning, and a game in which five stones were placed on the back of the hand, thrown upwards, and caught in the palm. One kind of game or exercise consisted in throwing a rope over a high post, when two boys took the ends of the rope, one boy on each side, the one trying to pull the other up. The most important exercises, however, were running, walking, throwing the discus, jumping, wrestling, boxing, and dancing.

The first public gymnasium in Rome was built by the Emperor Nero. In the time of the Republic Greek exercises were held in contempt by the Romans, and the first gymnasia in Rome were small, and connected only with private houses or villas.

The gymnasia were dedicated to Apollo, the god of healing, and exercises were considered of greater importance for restoring health than medicinal treatment. The directors of the gymnasia were in reality physicians, and acted as such. Plato states that one of these, Iccus by name, was the inventor of medical gymnastics. As in our own day, many creditable gymnasts, originally weak of body, had perfected their strength by systematic exercise and careful dieting.

Hippocrates had occasion to protest against prolonged and laborious exercises, and excessive massage, and recommended his own system, that of moderation. He applied massage to reduce swellings in suitable cases, and also recognized that the same treatment was capable of increasing nutrition, and of producing increased growth and development. Hippocrates described exercises of the kind now known as Swedish, consisting of free movements without resistance.

Galen generally followed the teaching of Hippocrates on gymnastics, and wrote a whole book on the merits of using the strigil. Oribasius, and Antyllus, too, in their writings, recommend special exercises which appealed to their judgment.

The ancient physicians had great faith in the efficacy of exercises in cases of dropsy, and Asclepiades employed this method of treatment very extensively, using also pleasant medicaments, so that Pliny said "this physician made himself the delight of mankind." Patients suffering from consumption were commonly sent to Alexandria to benefit from the climate, but Celsus considered the sea voyage most beneficial because the patient was exercised bodily by the motion of the ship. Germanicus was cured by riding exercise, and Cicero was strengthened by travelling and massage.

From the writings of Greek and Roman physicians there is no other conclusion to be drawn but that exercises and gymnastics were in great vogue for medical purposes, and were of the utmost benefit. It seems likely that the exercises of the Greeks, and the baths of the Romans, both freed from the abuses which took away in time from their merits, could be adopted at the present day and encouraged by physicians with great advantage to their patients. There is a strong tendency at present in that direction.

Belonging to a different class were the contests of the athletes, who, except in very early times in Greece, were people of the baser sort whose bodies were developed to the neglect of their minds. Those who underwent the severest training ate enormous quantities of meat, and tried to cultivate bulk and weight rather than strength. They did not compete, as a rule, after the age of thirty-five years. Euripides considered these athletes an encumbrance on the State. Plato said they were very subject to disease, without grace of manner, violent, and brutal. Aristotle declared that the athletes had not the active vigour that good citizens ought to possess.

The athletes and gladiators of Rome were mostly Greeks. Both Plutarch and Galen deride them. The former condemned the whole business, and Galen wrote six chapters to warn young men against becoming athletes. He said that man is linked to the divine and also to the lower animals, that the link with animals was developed by athletics, and that athletes were immoderate in eating, sleeping, and exertion, and were therefore unhealthy, and more liable than other people to disease and sudden death. Their brutal strength was of use only on rare occasions and unsuited for war, or for useful work.

In the time of St. Paul, the athletes were evidently abstemious, for he wrote "every man who striveth in the games is temperate in all things," but in Rome, at most periods of their history this class of men was notorious for grossness and brutality.

BATHS

Greek Baths.--In Greece from very early times inability to read and to swim were considered the marks of the ignorant. In Homer's time over-indulgence in warm baths was considered effeminate.[41] The system of bathing was never so complete in Greece as in Rome, but in the former country there were both public and private baths, and ancient Greek vases display pictures of swimming-baths and shower-baths, and also of large basins for men and for women round which they stood to bathe. The Greek baths were near the gymnasia. After the bath, the bathers were anointed with oil and took refreshments. Sometimes a material consisting of a lye made of lime or wood-ashes, of nitrum and of fuller's earth was applied to the body. Towels and strigils were employed for rubbing and scraping after the anointing; the strigil was, as a rule, made of iron.

Natural warm springs used for curative purposes are mentioned by ancient Greek writers.

Roman Baths.--Bathing, which was not much in vogue in Rome in the most ancient times, was more common during the Republic, and became a factor in the decay of the nation in the time of the Empire. Seneca informs us that the ancient Romans washed their arms and legs every day and their whole bodies once a week. The bath-room was near the kitchen in the Roman house, to be convenient for the supply of hot water. Scipio's bath was "small and dark after the manner of the ancients." In the time of Cicero, the use of baths, both public and private, was general, and hot-water and hot-air baths are both mentioned. It has been computed that there were 856 baths in Rome in the time of Constantine.

The public baths were at first used only by the poor, but the mother of Augustus went to the public bath, and in time even the emperors patronized them. The baths were opened at sunrise and closed at sunset except in the time of Alexander Severus, when they were open also at night. The charges for admission were very low. The ringing of a bell announced that the bath was ready. Baths were taken seven or eight times in succession when the people were given to luxury, and some of them wasted almost the whole day there. The voluptuaries of the Empire bathed not only before the principal meal of the day, but also afterwards to promote digestion as they thought. The perspiration induced by the bath took the place of honest sweat induced by work or exercise, and excessive hot-bathing and perspiring in some cases had a fatal ending.

Galen and Celsus differ in their directions to bathers. Galen recommended first the hot-air bath, next the hot-water bath, then the cold bath and finally rubbing; Celsus recommended sweating first in the tepid chamber, then in the hot chamber, and next the pouring of hot, then tepid, and lastly, cold water over the head, followed by the use of the strigil, and anointing and rubbing.

The plan of the baths at Pompeii, which was largely a pleasure resort, is typical of the public baths that were in general use. These baths had several entrances, and the principal one led to a covered portico from which a lavatory opened. The portico ran round three sides of a courtyard (atrium) in which the attendants waited, and it was also the exercise-yard for the young men. Advertisements of the theatres and gladiatorial shows were exhibited on the walls of the atrium. The undressing room was also the reception room and meeting-place. The bathers' garments were handed over for custody to slaves, who were, as a general rule, a very dishonest class. The frigidarium contained a cold bath 13 ft. 8 in. in diameter, and a little less than 4 ft. deep.

It had two marble steps, and a seat under water 10 in. from the bottom. Water ran into the bath through a bronze spout, and there was a conduit for the outflow, and an overflow pipe. The frigidarium opened into the tepidarium which was heated with hot air from furnaces, and furnished with a charcoal brazier and benches. The brazier at Pompeii was 7 ft. long and 2-1/2 ft. broad. The tepidarium was commonly a beautifully ornamented apartment, while the anointing-room was conveniently situated off it. Pliny has described the various unguents used by wealthy and luxurious Romans. From the tepidarium the bather might enter the caldarium or sweating room, an apartment constructed with double walls and floor, between which hot air was made to pass. This room contained a labrum, or circular marble basin, containing cold water for pouring over the head before the bather left the caldarium. The method of heating rooms by passing hot air between the "hanging" and the lower floor was in use in the better class of houses, and the device can at present be seen in some of the buildings on the Palatine Hill in Rome, and in the ruins of the great Baths of Caracalla. After a course of sweating the bather had the sweat removed from his body by the strigil, in much the same way as a horse is scraped with a bent piece of hoop-iron by a groom. The guttus was a small vessel with a narrow neck adapted for dropping oil on the strigil to lubricate its working edge. Pliny states that invalids used sponges instead of strigils. Rubbing with towels followed the use of the strigil, and the bather finally lounged in the tepidarium for a varying period before entering the outer air.

The boilers in use at Pompeii were three in number. The lowest one, immediately over the furnace, contained the hottest water. The next above and a short distance to the side held tepid water, and the farthest removed contained cold water. This system was economical because as the very hot water was drawn off from the lowest boiler a supply of tepid water flowed down from the boiler next above, and from the highest to the middle boiler.

A smaller suite of bathing apartments adjoining the men's establishment was for the use of women.

The most important baths formed only a part of the great establishments called therm? Adjoining the baths of the therm?were a gymnasium for sports and exercises, a library for the studious, lounging places for the idle, halls for poets and philosophers, in which they declaimed and lectured, museums of art, and sometimes shady groves. These complete establishments were first erected by Marcus Agrippa in the time of Augustus. Succeeding emperors vied with each other in providing magnificent therm? and the ruins of the Baths of Caracalla remain in a wonderful state of preservation to this day. The building of these baths began in A.D. 216. The structure, 1,050 ft. long and 1,390 ft. broad, was on a scale of almost incredible magnificence. Priceless statues and rare objects of art have been unearthed from the ruins. In recent years excavations have revealed a complicated system of subterranean corridors and galleries which existed for the purpose of carrying leaden water-pipes to the baths, and providing a passage-way for the host of slaves who acted as bath-attendants. The great buildings were well lit by windows in the walls of the courtyards, and these openings also allowed for ventilation. A great stadium and beautiful gardens adjoined the Baths of Caracalla. In the north-west section of these baths Alessio Valle has very recently discovered the remains of a great public library. When Caracalla pillaged Alexandria he probably carried off many of the books from the famous library there to enrich his baths. The ruins of the library in the Baths of Caracalla reveal circular tiers of galleries for the display of manuscripts and papyri. There were 500 rooms round these baths. The great hall had a ceiling made in one span, and the roof was an early example of reinforced concrete, for it was made of concrete in which bronze bars were laid. The lead for the water-pipes was probably brought from Cornwall.

The Therm?of Diocletian could accommodate 3,200 bathers. Its tepidarium was 300 ft. long by nearly 100 ft. wide, "vaulted in three bays with simple quadripartite groining, which springs from eight monolithic columns of Egyptian granite about 50 ft. high and 5 ft. in diameter" (Middleton).

From the medical point of view, these great bathing institutions were capable of being used for the treatment of various diseases, and for physical culture. No doubt, they were extensively employed for these purposes and with good results, but their legitimate use became increasingly limited, and abuse of them was a prime factor in promoting national decay. To show to what an extent luxurious bathing was carried in some instances, it is interesting to read that baths were taken sometimes in warm perfumes, in saffron oil, and that the voluptuous Poppel soothed her skin in baths of milk drawn from a herd of 500 she-asses.

FOOTNOTES:

[41] Od. viii, 249.

CHAPTER XIII.

SANITATION.

Water-supply--Its extent--The Aqueducts--Distribution in city--Drainage--Disposal of the Dead--Cremation and Burial--Catacombs--Public Health Regulations.

THE WATER-SUPPLY.

In ancient Greece, the cities were supplied with water from springs over which beautiful fountains were erected. The Greek aqueducts were not on the same grand scale as the Roman, but were usually rectangular channels cut in the rock, or made of pipes or masonry. Great care was taken in the supervision of these public works.

The first Roman aqueduct, according to Frontinus, dates from 312 B.C.

Pliny wrote of the Claudian aqueduct: "But if anyone will carefully calculate the quantity of the public supply of water, for baths, reservoirs, houses, trenches, gardens and suburban villas, and, along the distance which it traverses, the arches built, the mountains perforated, the valleys levelled, he will confess that there never was anything more wonderful in the whole world."

Frontinus, who was controller of the aqueducts in the time of Nerva and of Trajan, describes nine aqueducts, of which four belonged to the days of the Republic, and five to the reigns of Augustus and Claudius.

"The total water-supply of Rome has been estimated at 332,306,624 gallons a day, or, taking the population at a million, 332 gallons a head. Forty gallons a day is now considered sufficient."[42]

The ancient Aqua Virgo at the present day supplies the magnificent Fontana di Trevi, and the glorious fountains in the Piazzo di Spagna and the Piazzo Navona.

The Romans not only provided great aqueducts for the Imperial City, but also built them throughout various parts of the Empire. In Rome, the aqueducts were built to supply both the low and the high levels of the city. The reason why the Romans did not build underground aqueducts, as is done at the present day, has been variously explained. Perhaps they did not fully understand that water will find its own level over a great distance. They also would have found great difficulty in overcoming the high pressure of the water.

In their conduits they built shafts at frequent intervals designed to relieve the pressure of compressed air in the pipes. The water from the neighbourhood of Rome rapidly encrusted channels and pipes with calcareous deposits. Probably the great advantage of accessibility to leaks and defects gained by building unenclosed aqueducts appealed strongly to the ancient Romans. They did not fully understand the technical difficulties involved in the "hydraulic mean gradient." No machinery was used to pump the water or raise it to an artificial level. A strip of land 15 ft. wide was left on either side of the aqueducts, and this land was defined at intervals by boundary stones. No trees were grown near the aqueduct, to avoid the risk of injuring the foundations, and any breach of the rules for the preservation of the aqueducts was severely punished by fines.

Vitruvius gives rules for testing the water, and points out that water led through earthen pipes is more wholesome than water coming from leaden ones. He states that the "fall" of an aqueduct should be not less than 1 in 200. A circuit was often made to prevent the too rapid flow of the water, and intermediate reservoirs were constructed to avoid a shortage of water in the case of a broken main. Reservoirs were also used for irrigation.

The water from the aqueduct was received at the walls of the city in a great reservoir called castellum aquarum, externally a beautiful building and internally a vast chamber lined with hard cement and covered with a vaulted roof supported on pillars. The water flowed thence into three smaller reservoirs, the middle one filled by the overflow of the two outer ones. The outer reservoirs supplied the public baths and private houses, while the middle one supplied the public ponds and fountains, so that, in the event of a shortage of water, the first supply to fail was the least important. The amount of water provided for private use could be checked, for purposes of revenue, by means of this arrangement.

At first the aqueducts were not connected with private houses, but, later, private persons were allowed to buy the water which escaped from leaks in the aqueducts. Next, private connections were made with the public mains, and, finally, reservoirs were built at the expense of adjoining households, but these reservoirs, although built with private money, were considered part of the public property. Water rights were renewed with each change of occupant. The water-supply to a house was measured by the size of the pipe through which it passed at the in-flow and at the out-flow of the reservoir.

The curatores aquarum had very responsible duties. Under their orders, in the time of Trajan, were 460 slaves who were subdivided into various classes, each of which had its own particular duties to perform in connection with the maintenance and control of the water-supply. A supply of pure water and proper drainage are of first importance in sanitation, and it is evident that the Romans understood these matters well.

DRAINAGE.

The drains of Athens, built of brick and stone and provided with air-shafts, ran into a basin from which pipes carried the sewage beneath the surrounding plain which it helped to fertilize.

The chief drain of Rome was the Cloaca Maxima, and there was a great network of smaller drains. The privy in private houses was usually situated near the kitchen, and a common drain from the kitchen and the privy discharged into the public cloaca. A pipe opened just above the floor of the closet to supply water for flushing. Ruins of very small rooms have been discovered in the Via Sacra of the Roman Forum, and it has puzzled archeologists to discover their use, but they are thought to have been sanitary closets. The sewers of Rome drained into the Tiber.

DISPOSAL OF THE DEAD.

Both in Greece and Rome earth-burial and cremation were employed for the disposal of the dead. Near the Temple of Faustina in the Roman Forum, under the Via Sacra, have been found the graves of some of the dwellers of the hills before Romulus founded the city. In Rome, burial within the city was forbidden from the time of the Twelve Tables. Exceptions were made in the case of emperors, vestal virgins, and famous men, such as those who had been honoured with triumphs. The large cemetery for the poor lay on the east side of the city and the tombs of the rich were along the roadsides. The remains of some of these can now be seen along the Appian Way. One of these tombs is the Tomb of the Scipios, which, as Byron wrote, "contains no ashes now." Near the Tomb of the Scipios can be seen a door with high steps which leads to the columbaria. These are little rooms provided with pigeon-holes for the reception of the ashes of the freedmen of notabilities. Inscriptions show that some of these freedmen were physicians, and others musicians and silversmiths. The shops of the perfumers stood in a part of the Forum on the Via Sacra. Perfumes were much used at incinerations to disguise the smell of decomposition before the fires were kindled. The Christians opposed cremation and favoured earth burial, and in time the business of the perfume-sellers failed, and Constantine bought their shops.

The Catacombs were used almost entirely by the Christians. If all the passages of the Catacombs could be placed in line, it is said that they would extend the whole length of Italy. They were hewn out of volcanic soil very well suited for the purpose, and were probably extensions, in the first place, of quarries made for the purpose of obtaining building cement. They were used by the Christians, not only for the religious rite of burial, but also as secluded meeting places. The bodies were laid in loculi, sometimes in two or three tiers, the loculi being filled in with earth and stone.

Many of our public health regulations had their counterpart in ancient times, for instance, any factory or workshop in Rome which created a public nuisance had to be removed outside the city. The spoliarium of the Coliseum was an ancient morgue.

A detached building or room, valetudinarium, was provided in large houses for sick slaves. This was for the purpose of preventing infection as well as for convenient attendance on the sick.

FOOTNOTES:

[42] "Dict. of Gr. and Rom. Antiq.," Smith, vol. i, p. 150, to which the author is indebted for much of the information herein supplied.

APPENDIX.

FEES IN ANCIENT TIMES.

The professional incomes of doctors in ancient Greece and Rome varied greatly as at the present day. A few were paid very large fees, but the rank and file did not make more money than was equal to keeping them in decency.

Seleucus paid Erasistratus about ?0,000 for curing his son Antiochus. Herodotus mentions that they paid Democedes, from the public treasury, ?04 a year; the Athenians afterwards paid him ?06 a year, and at Samos he received ?22 yearly. Pliny says that Albutius, Arruntius, Calpetanus, Cassius and Rubrius each made close upon ?,000 a year, and that Quintus Stertinius favoured the Emperor by accepting about ?,000 a year when he could have made more in private practice. The surgeon Alcon made a fortune of nearly ?00,000 by a few years' practice in Gaul. Pliny states that Manlius Cornutus paid his doctor ?,000 for curing him of a skin disease, and Galen's fee for curing the wife of a consul was about ?00 of our money.

www.ingramcontent.com/pod-product-compliance
Lightning Source LLC
Chambersburg PA
CBHW070325190526
45169CB00005B/1750